BIOMEDICAL & NANOMEDICAL TECHNOLOGIES
CONCISE MONOGRAPH SERIES

Magnetic Bearings for Mechanical Cardiac Assist Devices

Steven Day

Shanbao Cheng

Arnold David Gomez

Co-published by Momentum Press, LLC, 222 E. 46th Street, #203, New York, NY 10017, USA (www.momentumpress.net)

Library of Congress Cataloging-in-Publication Data

Names: Day, Steven (Steven W.) author. | Cheng, Shanbao author. | Gomez, Arnold David author.
Title: Magnetic bearings for assist devices / Steven Day, Shanbao, Cheng Arnold David Gomez.
Description: New York, NY : ASME Press, [2015]
Identifiers: LCCN 2015037208 | ISBN 9780791860410
Subjects: LCSH: Biomedical materials. | Magnetic bearings. | Cardiovascular instruments, Implanted. | Medical technology.
Classification: LCC R857.M3 D39 2015 | DDC 610.28--dc23 LC record available at http://lccn.loc.gov/2015037208

Print ISBN: 978-0-7918-60410

ASME Order No. 860410

Electronic ISBN: 9781606509203

Guest Editors' Preface

According to the American Heart Association, approximately 5 million Americans have congestive heart failure (CHF) and more than half a million new cases are reported every year. CHF is a chronic condition in which at least one chamber of the heart is not pumping well enough to meet the body's need. Heart failure presents an increasing public burden of morbidity and mortality even as the mortality from coronary artery disease and hypertension is decreasing. It is estimated that at least 40,000 of these patients are candidates for heart transplantation; however, only 3,800 donor hearts are made available each year worldwide. While effective pharmacologic therapies have improved outcomes for mild to moderate CHF, the need for mechanical circulatory support is well defined and growing.

Current use of mechanical circulatory cardiac devices is dominated by the indications of post-cardiotomy shock and bridging to transplantation. About 6,000 patients a year receive support devices after cardiac surgery, in the U.S. alone. However, most of the devices do not allow for hospital discharge of patients. If fully implantable and wearable devices were available, at least 100,000 patients annually could benefit from this technology.

Significant technological advances have been made in the past thirty years in the design and development of mechanical cardiac circulatory support devices. Several recent review articles and book chapters have summarized the state-of-the-art in this critical medical technology. However, a comprehensive and focused publication on this subject is currently lacking. The comprehensive review articles in this concise monograph series have been written by an international team of experts with many years of experience in design of mechanical cardiovascular assist devices and performance evaluation, both in pre-clinical and clinical testing, as well as issues related to standards and regulatory requirements.

Said Jahanmir
William J. Weiss
Conrad M. Zapanta

Series Editors' Preface

Biomedical and Nanomedical Technologies (B&NT)
This **concise** monograph series focuses on the implementation of various engineering principles in the conception, design, development, analysis and operation of biomedical, biotechnological and nanotechnology systems and applications. The primary objective of the series is to compile the latest research topics in biomedical and nanomedical technologies, specifically devices and materials.

Each volume comprises a collection of invited manuscripts, written in an accessible manner and of a concise and manageable length. These timely collections will provide an invaluable resource for initial enquiries about technologies, encapsulating the latest developments and applications with reference sources for further detailed information. The content and format have been specifically designed to stimulate further advances and applications of these technologies by reaching out to the non-specialist across a broad audience.

Contributions to *Biomedical and Nanomedical Technologies* will inspire interest in further research and development using these technologies and encourage other potential applications. This will foster the advancement of biomedical and nanomedical applications, ultimately improving healthcare delivery.

Editor:
Ahmed Al-Jumaily, PhD, Professor of Biomechanical Engineering & Director of the Institute of Biomedical Technologies, Auckland University of Technology.

Associate Editors:
Christopher H.M. Jenkins, PhD, PE, Professor and Head, Mechanical & Industrial Engineering Department, Montana State University.

Said Jahanmir, PhD, President and CEO, Boston Tribology Associates.

Shanzhong (Shawn) Duan, PhD, Professor, Mechanical Engineering, South Dakota State University.

Conrad M. Zapanta, PhD, Associate Department Head of Biomedical Engineering, Teaching Professor of Biomedical Engineering, Carnegie Mellon University.

William J. Weiss, PhD, Professor of Surgery and Bioengineering, College of Medicine, The Pennsylvania State University.

Siddiq M. Qidwai, PhD, Mechanical Engineer, U.S. Naval Research Laboratory.

Table of Contents

Abstract

Magnetic bearings are mechatronic devices that produce contact-free electromagnetic force to support a load, such as a moving train or a spinning rotor. Compared to traditional bearings, magnetic bearings offer several advantages: no friction, low heat generation, no required lubrication, quiet operation, and fast and stable rotation. Because of these reasons, magnetic bearings have been used in rotary ventricular assist devices (VADs) to increase design life, reduce or eliminate material wear and bearing maintenance, as well as to increase biocompatibility by eliminating high fluid stresses and heat generation, both of which are associated with hemolysis, platelet activation and aggregation, and thrombus growth.

In this chapter, magnetic bearings and their application in VADs are introduced. First, the operating principles of magnetic bearings are introduced. Typical structures of passive bearings, which are comprised solely of permanent magnets, and active magnetic bearings (AMB), which make use of electromagnets and position sensors to control the position of the rotor, are described. We include some description of all the components of a typical AMB system, including actuator, position sensor, controller, and amplifier, as well as different structures of electromagnet actuators, coils design, and iron selection. A range of position sensors, including those typically used in blood pumps, as well as self-sensing bearings are discussed. The basics of the hardware and the software (control laws) that comprise a typical magnetic bearing system are described. A section describes the performance considerations of magnetic bearings and the effect on the overall performance of an assist device that uses magnetic bearings. Lastly, the magnetic suspension of existing VADs with magnetic bearings are described: Berlin Heart INCOR, Heartware HVAD, WorldHeart Levacor and MiFlow, Terumo Duraheart, PediaFlow, MiTiHeart, and LEV-VAD.

1 Magnetic bearings for assist devices

Magnetic bearings produce contact-free electromagnetic force to stably support rotors or other loads. Compared to traditional bearings, magnetic bearings offer the advantages of no friction, low heat generation, no required lubrication, quiet operation, and fast and stable rotation. Because of these reasons, magnetic bearings have been used in rotary ventricular assist devices (VADs) in order to increase design life, reduce or eliminate material wear and bearing maintenance, as well as to increase biocompatibility by eliminating high fluid stresses and heat generation, both of which have been associated with hemolysis, platelet activation, and thrombus growth. Magnetic bearings have been used in several of the most recently developed mechanical circulatory assist devices as a means to extend pump life. This includes extending the mechanical life of the pump by eliminating material wear, but also minimizing damage of red blood cells and other blood factors and the formation of blood clots, both of which are physiological phenomena associated with elevated fluid shear stress and heat generation.

The advantages of magnetic bearings have been proven in other applications such as high-speed trains [1, 2] and turbomachinery [3–5]. Advanced magnetic bearings have benefited from recent significant developments of enabling technologies, including novel materials capable of strong magnetic forces and small, fast, and affordable digital computers. These are critical to supporting high speed rotating elements, such as pump impellers, because relatively large magnetic forces have to be applied at very precise times. Fully magnetically levitated (Mag-Lev) ventricular assist pumps are more recent developments, having grown in the last ten years [6–12]. Control of blood pumps poses interesting challenges, including position sensing and control through blood-tight enclosures, and robustness to electromagnetic and mechanic disturbances. Additionally, the high forces inherent to these small sized systems creates high instability, which in turn generates a need to read, process, and actuate multiple channels at high sampling rates. Nonetheless, a variety of academic and corporate research groups have produced a range of Mag-Lev pumps ranging from axial [13–16] to mixed flow to centrifugal [17] configurations, from early bench-top testing to clinical use, and that vary widely in size and magnetic configuration [18].

This chapter provides a brief summary of magnetic bearings and their application in VADs. First, the operation principles of the magnetic bearings are introduced in Section 1. Typical structures of passive bearings, which are comprised solely of permanent magnets, and active magnetic bearings, which make use of electromagnets to control the position of the rotor/impeller via position sensors with feedback control, are described. All the components of an AMB system, including actuator, position sensor, amplifiers, and control laws, are introduced and described in some detail in this chapter. A section describes the performance considerations of magnetic bearings and the effect on the overall performance of an assist device that uses magnetic bearings. Lastly, the magnetic suspension of existing VADs with magnetic bearings are described: Berlin Heart INCOR, Heartware HVAD, WorldHeart Levacor, Terumo Duraheart, PediaFlow, MiTiHeart, and LEV-VAD.

1.1 Fundamentals of magnetic bearings

In the most general form, a magnetic bearing is composed of two components with relative motion with respect to each other. One component is stationary whereas the other levitates and is able to move in a controlled manner. In the case of rotating machinery, these components are concentric. In this chapter, we will refer to the stationary and moving parts as the pump stator and rotor, respectively. In principle, a force acts between materials if there is a magnetic flux between them. Magnetic flux may be generated by permanent or electromagnets and may pass through nonmagnetic materials, such as air, conduits, or blood, and may be guided by paramagnetic materials, such as iron. The force of the magnetic flux on any of the components depends on the magnetic permeability of the material, the intensity of the flux and the area over which the flux is distributed.

A simple horseshoe magnet and a piece of steel have a flux and resultant force, but they do not constitute a bearing because they are attracted to one another until they touch. The two objects are not generating forces that would repel each other, which would be necessary for levitation. A magnetic bearing must exert a force that keeps two objects at a non-zero distance from one another, as illustrated in Figure 1 for a concentric radial bearing.

Along a single axis of motion, a bearing can operate either passively, using permanent magnets to generate flux and a resultant force, or actively, using electromagnets for flux and resultant force generation. The flux and resultant force from a passive bearing of some given geometry

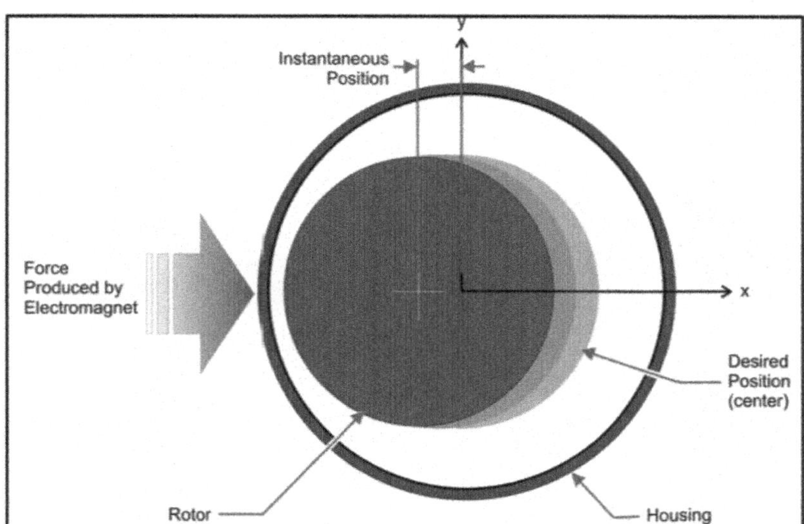

Figure 1 Schematic of the desired function of a radial magnetic bearing: Ideally, the rotor is centered within the stator (or housing) by electromagnetic forces.

and materials is a function of the relative position of rotor and stator. If there is no active control, as is the case for the active case, a passive bearing assembly that is passively stable in any coordinate direction will be unstable in at least one orthogonal direction. Then, additional active control forces are necessary to stabilize the rotor. For example, the bearing shown in Figure 1 is radially stable (against displacements in the x or y direction) if the there are forces pushing the rotor back towards radial center that effectively keep the rotor radially centered within the stator housing. However, it a passive axial force can be used to stabilize the out-of-plane direction. It is often convenient to assign a global coordinate system to strategize the selection and implementation for a magnetic levitation approach. A magnetic bearing rotor test assembly and its respective the degrees of freedom (DOF) with respect to a global coordinate system are shown in Figure 2.

1.1.1 Considerations of a full magnetic suspension

The motion of a rotor or other levitating object can be described in 6 degrees of freedom (three translational along x, y, and z direction and three rotational movements about these same axes), as shown in Figure 2. One might strategize to simply add more bearing components to

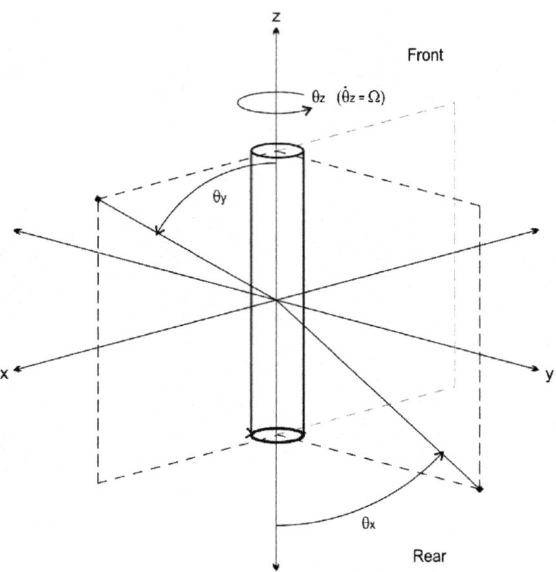

Figure 2   Coordinate system showing the rotor's six degrees of freedom (DOF): In an axial pump, the speed (rate of change of Θz) is controlled by the motor. The remaining five DOF are controlled by the magnetic bearing system.

the system to force stability in the unstable direction. Unfortunately, these additional components introduce instability in their orthogonal directions so that the system remains passively unstable. It has been shown for some time that a body cannot be held in stable equilibrium by electrostatic forces from other charged bodies [19] and this extends to passive magnetic bearings and systems of passive magnetic bearings. A system of combined magnetic bearings may be designed to make up to 5 DOF passively stable, but any system of combined passive bearing components cannot be passively stable in all degrees of freedom. At a minimum, one degree of freedom will require some other means of stabilization.

A popular gift shop toy, Figure 3, demonstrates the need of an additional non-electrostatic force to suspend a rotor in an arrangement akin to the rotor shown in Figure 2. The rotor is passively levitated in radial directions and for rotations θx and θy about these axes. In this implementation, it is also free to spin about the longitudinal axis (labeled z) due to homopolar bearings (they are symmetric about their z axis), but

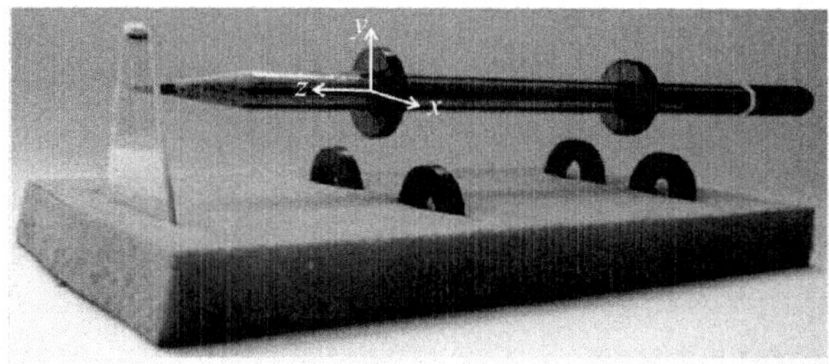

Figure 3 Simple toy demonstrating nearly full magnetic levitation using only permanent magnets: The rotor is free to rotate. Four degrees of freedom are held stable by magnets, but the axial motion is constrained by a mechanical reaction force from the clear wall shown at the left. From: http://www.arvindguptatoys.com.

it unstable in the axial direction. There is one axial location that corresponds to zero force on the rotor, but if it is displaced axially from this location, the magnetic bearing system pushes the rotor further in the same axial direction. In the toy, this unstable DOF is stabilized only by the presence of the clear plastic wall shown in the figure, which exerts a mechanical force onto the rotor. The magnetic forces are continually trying to push the rotor into the wall. This force may be felt by moving the impeller a very small distance away from the wall. If the rotor is pulled further from the wall, it passes the point of neutral force and the bearing system will act to push the rotor even further away, at which point it will fall out of suspension. As the rotor moves even further axially, the radial bearings lose force capacity and the system falls.

In the end, some force, other than passive magnetic force must be used to maintain stability in at least one degree of freedom. This can be done mechanically (as the gift shop toy in Figure 3), hydrodynamically, or with an actively controlled magnetic bearing, as will be the primary topic of this chapter. In a pump, rotor suspension is an extension of the same basic approach. Additional design variations, as well as other design considerations are presented later in the chapter.

1.1.2 Active magnetic bearing (AMB)

Aside from combined magnetic and hydrodynamic systems, all bearing systems that fully suspend a rotor contain as least one active magnetic bearing (AMB). In the generic AMB system, shown schematically in

Figure 4. Essential components include a position sensor to measure the position of the levitated object and transmit this information to a controller that determines the appropriate control effort. An amplifier then transforms this control effort into a control current, which powers an actuator whose output force is a function of this controller current. This chapter is organized to discuss each of these components: actuators, position sensors, and controllers individually in the following sections.

In practice, the actuators and sensors that are contained within the pump may require additional intermediate electronics to interface with the controller. Actuators are high current devices that require amplifiers, and some signal conditioning of the position sensors is usually required for the sensors. An additional data acquisition system is typically used to monitor the bearing performance, including position sensor data and actuator effort. This is necessary in prototyping and may serve

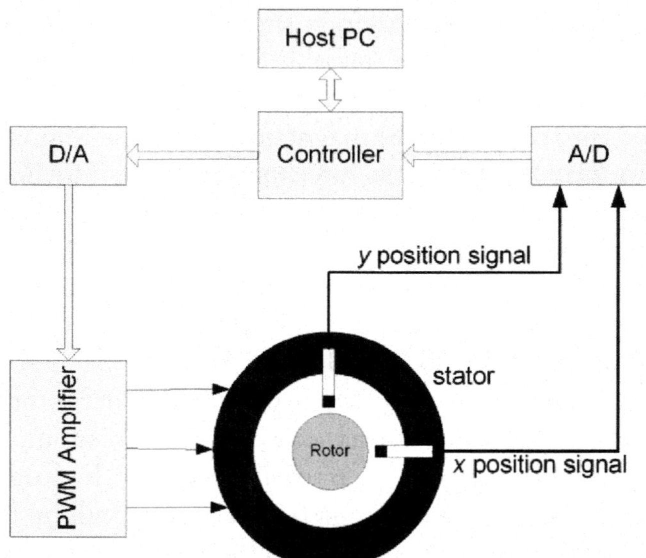

Figure 4 Active Magnetic Bearing (AMB) schematic: The essential components include a controller, analog to digital converters (ADC), the magnetic bearing, sensors and amplifiers. This configuration uses pulse width modulation (PWM) to drive the system, and a host computer was added to record information and to update the controller's software.

diagnostic purposes even during normal use. Figure 5 shows a typical schematic of the physical components required to operate and study a magnetic levitation system. The controller, amplifiers, power supply, and pump prototype are the essential functional components, which would be reduced to circuit boards and micro-processors in a clinical device. The monitoring system is not controlling the magnetic bearings, but is recording or relaying information about the entire system.

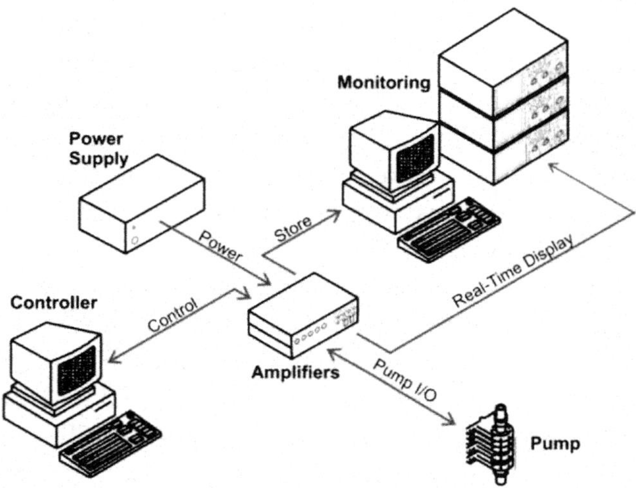

Figure 5 Typical experimental setup of a magnetic levitation system: The arrows denote physical connections.

2 Structure of magnetic actuator

2.1 Properties of magnetic materials

Magnetic susceptibility is a fundamental material property that determines the net behavior of a material in the presence of a magnetic field, and it is responsible for the colloquial descriptions of being *magnetic* or *non-magnetic* depending on whether or not the material will be attracted to a magnet. More specifically, a material's magnetic behavior can be classifies as: paramagnetic, diamagnetic, or ferromagnetic. Materials with positive magnetic susceptibility are called paramagnetic, and will be weakly attracted to permanent magnets. The opposite is true of diamagnetic materials, which have negative magnetic susceptibility. Most commonly, ferromagnetic materials, like iron, are known commonly as being *magnetic*, and if a substance has magnetic susceptibility near zero, it is said to be *non-magnetic.*

Ferromagnetic materials will be attracted to permanent magnets because of molecular reconfiguration. To some extent, the magnitude of the attractive force is proportional to the strength of the permanent magnet, but the magnitude of this force is associated with the material's magnetic permeability. Materials with high permeability, such as iron, have high configuration, and therefore a high and positive susceptibility. Magnetic flux passes very easily through these materials and they would, therefore, be more strongly attracted to a permanent magnet than a material with low permeability.

Although all of the materials above have varying permeability to magnetic flux, they do not generate flux in the absence of an external magnetic field. Some materials, i.e., ferromagnetic materials, possess the ability to reconfigure under an external magnetic field and are able to keep a field of their own after the external influence is removed, which gives rise to permanent magnets.

2.2 Passive actuators

2.2.1 Typical passive configuration (radial passive bearing)

In general, dissimilar poles of a permanent magnet are attracted to one another and similar poles are repelled from one another. A structure as simple as two axially polarized ring magnets placed within one another could constitute a simple magnetic bearing. In the configuration shown in Figure 6, axial stability is the result of attraction between opposite

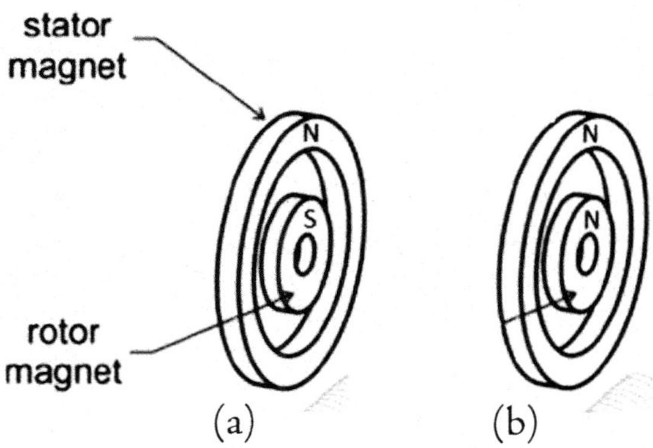

Figure 6 Examples of passive magnetic bearings: Simple axial bearings (a) and radial bearings (b) can be stacked into more complex configurations. In the figure, the N or S indicates the polarity of the right face of each ring magnet, which is visible in the figure. All magnets are polarized axially, so that the left facing (hidden) face is of the opposite polarity.

poles of the rotor and stator permanent magnetic bearings, which occurs due to a closed magnetic flux loop. Heuristically speaking, this flux loop is the lowest resistance when the rotor and stator are axially aligned. If the rotor were to be displaced in the z direction, the flux path would have a larger air gap and higher resistance. The system acts to restore a path of least resistance, so the system would act to pull the rotor back into axial alignment. Put another way, dissimilar N (north) and S (south) poles would act to pull themselves towards one another, realigning the rotor axially.

The force capacity of passive bearing configurations like this is fairly well understood and some recent publications have been dedicated to formulae that may be used for [20]. For a given configuration of magnets, the force is a function of displacement because variations in the air gap act to modulate the intensity of the flux loop. This force is, therefore, not controllable by an external means.

2.3 Active actuators

2.3.1 Typical radial configuration
The flux loop through the rotor and stator can also include an electromagnet so the magnitude of flux, and therefore attractive force, may be

modulated by varying the current passing through the electromagnet's coil. In all configurations, this electromagnet is located within the stator because of the practical consideration of needing wires connected to this component. In the simplest configuration, an electromagnet with permeable core is located within the stator and the corresponding rotor component is a permeable material.

The force between the components is a function of the magnetic flux intensity in the air gap between rotor and stator as well as the cross sectional area of the flux path as is crosses the air gap. It should be noted that, in practice, the *air gap* contains other materials including electrical isolation and other packaging materials, that may interfere with the theoretical force generation. Because the magnetic flux is generated by an electromagnet, the force of the actuator is given as

$$F = \frac{\mu_0 n^2 I^2 A_g}{4g^2} \tag{1}$$

where, μ_0 is the magnetic permeability of the air, n is the number of coil turns, I is the coil current, A_g is the pole face area (cross-sectional area of the flux path from rotor to stator), and g is the air gap distance between the electromagnet and the rotor. In the configuration shown in Figure 7, stability is achieved with control forces created by altering the net magnetic flux density in the two perpendicular radial components. In each component, flux density depends on the current passing through the electromagnet coils, so that by controlling the current flowing through the electromagnet, it is possible to generate control forces according to Equation 1. If the rotor is a magnetically susceptible material, but not

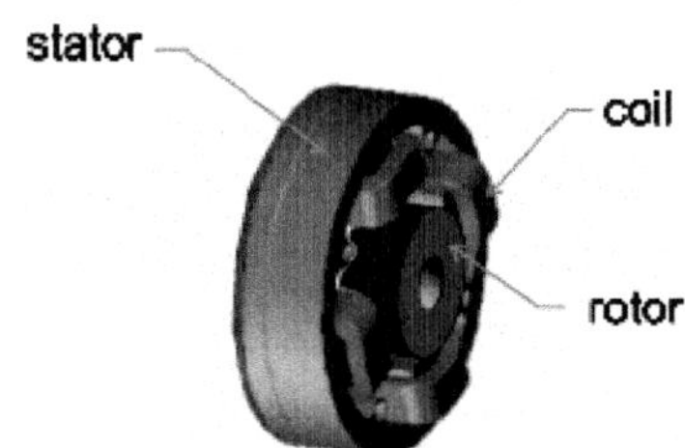

Figure 7 Typical configuration of an electromagnetic actuator: Current passes through the coils generating the forces used to center the rotor within the stator.

itself a permanent magnet, the magnet can only be used to attract the rotor, so a pair of opposed electromagnets, each actuated independently would be used to exert force in both directions. In theory, because rotor components are cylindrical, forces do not vary as a function of the rotational position of the rotor.

2.3.2 Flux biased magnetic bearings

Magnetic bearing systems are generally nonlinear, not only by the force-current relationship in Equation 1, but also from saturation and the so-called "dead zone" (i.e., current thresholds below which no force is exerted) effects. It is possible to operate the bearings assuming linearity within an operating range, and two opposing actuators may be used to minimize the effect of a dead zone through the application of a bias flux. Flux biasing may be achieved either by applying a biasing current, or with a permanent magnet as shown in Figure 8. In homopolar-type bearings (where the relative polarity between rotor and stator is unaffected by rotational position), flux biasing results from using a non-zero current at all times according to the resulting current-force calibration. In heteropolar-type bearings bias force must change direction according to the changes in polarity resulting from rotation. A permanent biasing magnet can be oriented in many different configurations, so long as the polarity of the magnet aligns with the desired flux path [21, 22]. Permanent-magnet-biased magnetic bearings can save energy by eliminating the bias current and are more efficient

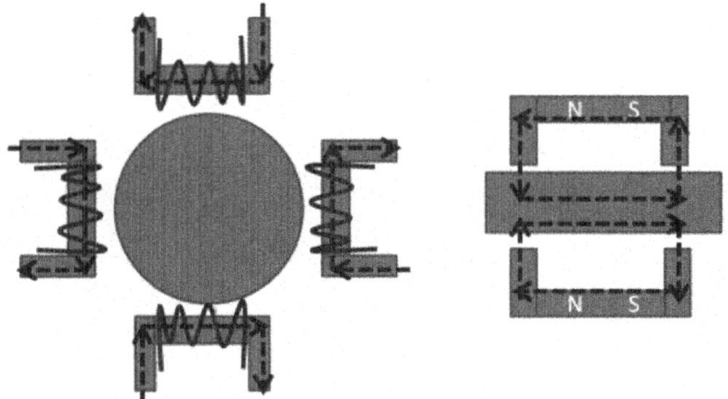

Figure 8 Biased magnetic bearing configurations: The dotted lines represent flux paths in current flux (left) and permanent magnet (right).

compared to current-biased magnetic bearings. For radial or axial magnetic bearings, current-biased magnetic bearings are usually smaller than permanent-magnet-biased magnetic bearings, because the latter need permanent magnets. Permanent-magnet-biased magnetic bearings allow for higher speed operations, and a stiffer, more robust shaft compared to current flux biased magnetic bearings, and therefore have become popular in industrial magnetic bearings. Due to the promise of increased efficiency and compact size, control strategies without magnetic flux biasing have been proposed and continue to be investigated [23].

2.4 Typical configuration of hybrid actuators

Single structure magnet designed to exert radial and axial forces, as well as to include passive and active electromagnetic elements. The schematic of a Hybrid Magnetic Bearing (HMB) is shown Figure 9. Flux distribution lines appear in Figure 10. Both the stator and rotor are composed of permanent magnets and ferromagnetic elements that guide the magnetic flux and act as the core of the electromagnet coils. As is the case for all bearings, active control is needed for at least one degree of freedom. In this particular bearing, the axial direction is passive and the radial is active [24]. Axial stability is the result of attraction between opposite poles of the rotor and stator permanent magnetic bearings, which occurs due to a

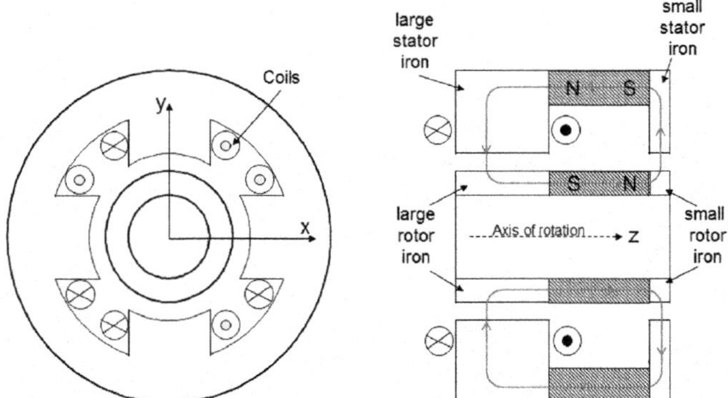

Figure 9   Potential configuration of a hybrid magnetic bearing passively stable in the axial direction: The same set of permanent magnets provides flux bias to the radial electromagnets. Left: Axial cross-section of the bearing; the x and y arrows define to the radial degrees of freedom. Right: orthogonal view where axial displacement is indicated by the z-axis.

closed magnetic flux loop very similar to the mechanism described for the simple bearing in Figure 6(a).

This same pair of permanent magnets acts to provide bias flux to the radial electromagnets, which are radially unstable passively as the N to S attraction would act to pull the rotor towards stator wall. The radial symmetry of the bearing makes is so that there is zero net force on the rotor when perfectly centered, but the attractive forces are amplified by proximity, so any radial displacement leads to increased forces in the same direction of the displacement and the system is inherently unstable. Radial suspension can only be achieved using forces caused by electromagnets distributed around the rotor. This is accomplished by controlling the electric current traveling through the coils, thus varying the magnetic flux, and generating forces along the x and y-axes in a controlled way.

In the general case of an actuator with both permanent magnet and electromagnetic components, the electromagnetic force F applied to the rotor can be expressed as a function of control current i and rotor displacement s:

$$F(i, s)_d = \kappa_d i_d - K_d s_d \qquad d = x, y, z \qquad (2)$$

where κ_d is the force-current factor (referred to here as *current stiffness*) and K_d is the force-displacement factor (also referred to as *position stiffness, radial or axial stiffness*). Each term has a subscript d to denote the direction as a bearing typically has different characteristics in each coordinate direction. The first term on the right hand side represents a force proportional to the electrical current through the coil and the second the passive magnetic force due to the rotor displacement and permanent magnet components of the bearing. There is a radial and axial component to both stiffness and displacement. In the particular bearing configuration shown in Figure 10, the axial component, K_z has a positive sign (like a spring), so that the bearing is inherently stable in this direction, but the radial components K_x and K_y have a negative sign, so that the suspension is unstable when operated radially in an open loop configuration. This system requires no control to remain stable in the axial direction, but requires active control with feedback to achieve system stability in the radial direction, and thus provide for complete magnetic levitation.

The maximum force exerted by a bearing is typically limited by the flux through the materials and the actuator cross-sectional area per

Equation 1. Some material properties, such as magnetic susceptibility and permeability play a significant role in determining the maximum flux. Other factors include: the area of the "foot" of the electromagnet, the maximum current that the electromagnet coils can conduct, and its number of turns. All these factors will affect design decisions, for example thicker wire or more turns will increase the bearing force, but will result in a bulkier bearing. We proceed to discuss some of these factors in the next two sections.

2.5 Electromagnetic coils

The induced magnetic field flux density in an electromagnet is a function of the square of the number of turns of the coil and the current through the wires, so increased number of turns leads to a stronger electromagnetic forces, but will increase the overall size of the bearings. Although they are shown schematically as simple circles in Figure 10,

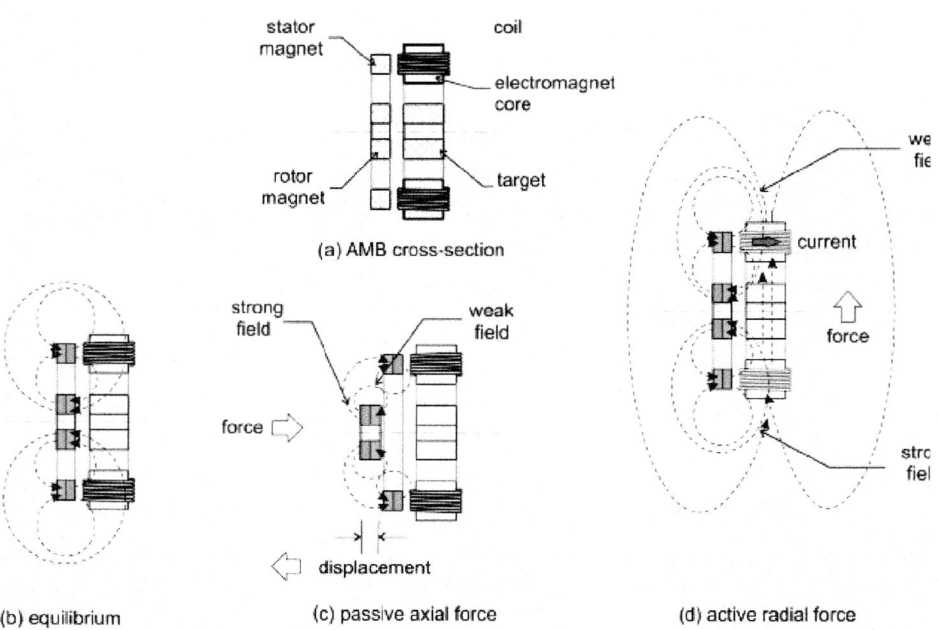

Figure 10 Functional description of hybrid magnetic bearing passively stable in the axial direction: (a) main components (b) flux paths (dotted lines) at equilibrium (c) axial stability via passive magnets (d) radial stability via active electromagnetic components.

the coils of an active bearing nearly fill the space between iron "legs". It is possible to use thinner wires to accommodate more turns in the same mass, but a thinner wire is less capable of conducting current. Alternative wire cross-section, such as "flat" or square, may improve the packing of turns into the same volume, or facilitate the construction of the electromagnet.

The current carrying capacity of copper is about 2×10^7 Amps/m^2. In practice, standard rules of current carrying capacity use gauge as a measure of diameter. Typical blood pump bearings and motors use less than an amp, which means that wire gauge 22 and up (only a few hundredths of an inch in diameter) is able to carry the load safely. Some actuator coils may use even lower currents. The typical construction of coil wire includes the conductor core, usually made of solid copper, and a thin insulation coating. This outer coating is designed to resist friction encountered during assembly and heat generated during operation, and to keep the coils electrically insulated at close proximity once wrapped in the coil. Additional chemicals, such as silicone or epoxy may be used for additional mechanical durability, thermal conductivity, and electrical isolation.

The wire coils that act to feed the flux loop can be placed most anywhere so long as they are wrapped around the iron that includes the flux path. Coils may be wound directly onto the stator, or onto a jig and subsequently assembled into their positon within the stator. Though it may be possible to include more windings, and achieve a more elaborate coil, by directly winding wire onto the stator leg one at the time by hand, this may not be efficient for high throughput. Alternatively, one can use prefabricated coils that are shaped to fit onto individual stator legs. In this case a coil is wound, then shaped according to the stator geometry using different forming techniques, such as pressing against a die.

Electrical connections of electromagnets have inherent design and manufacturing challenges given the need for mechanical robustness, low resistance between the connector and the coil, isolation from the conductor to the surroundings, and a small overall size of all components. The design of stator and other packaging components must include adequate clearances for wiring, and interconnections, while keeping a small size. Different levels of strain relief are needed so that the (usually thin) wires do not break during assembly or usage. The electrical connections may be soldered, crimped, or a combination of techniques. The connection may be coated with insulating chemicals, such as medical grade adhesives or silicones. Miniature connectors, when properly used, may facilitate the overall assembly of the device.

2.6 System configurations

The fundamental principles of magnetic bearings can be applied in a variety of configurations to support pumps with a rotating impeller. Some of these arrangements rely fully on the magnetic bearing system, whereas others only use magnetic means to stabilize some degrees of freedom. Bearing alternatives could include mechanical pivot bearings, or designing some fluidic components, such as the impeller and the driving motor, to help maintain rotor stability by hydrodynamic forces.

2.6.1 Centrifugal vs. axial-flow configurations

There are fundamentally two configurations of rotary turbomachines, axial flow and centrifugal flow, which are defined based on the orientation by which flow enters and leaves the pump relative to the axis of rotation, Figure 11. So-called mixed flow, or diagonal flow, pumps are intermediates between these two extremes. This overall topology can affect the magnetic bearing configuration because every actuator, as well as the motor, must have some components within the rotor and some within the stator. The effectiveness of any actuator is a function of, among other things, the size and distance between components. Equation 1 shows that the force capacity of a magnetic bearing decreases drastically as the air gap (distance between magnetic components in the rotor and the housing) increases.

Taken alone, this would certainly lead a designer to minimize this gaps between the rotor and the pump housing. However, in magnetically levitated blood pumps, the space between the stator and rotor is always filled with blood and this imposes a constraint on the minimum

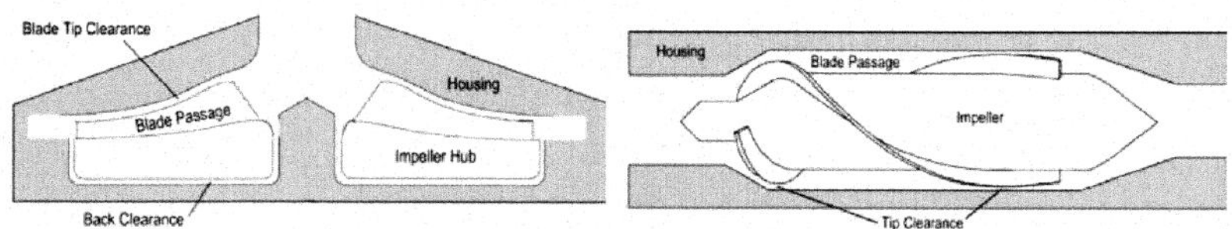

Figure 11 General configuration of centrifugal (left) and axial (right) flow pumps: Rotor components appear in white, and stator in grey.

distance between magnetic components. Within this space, one must provide enough space for the blood to flow between rotor and stator, biocompatible packaging of the magnetic components, and some mechanical clearance between the rotor and the housing. In some pumps, this magnetic gap is large enough to allow the rotor blades to be located and the magnets act through the primary blood path. In other pumps, the magnets are placed in areas other than the blade passages (secondary clearances) and can be made smaller because of this. Typically, magnetic air gaps (when filled with blood) are between 1 and 3mm in blood pumps, which is larger than the magnetic gap for most applications that don't have requirements related to blood passages and low shear stress.

The axial configuration, such as the PediaFlow [25], LEV-VAD [26], and mVAD [27] tend to rely on concentric elements, similar to the simple ring within ring bearing shown in Figure 6. The generated forces act through the primary blood path, which may increase the air gap, but which has the advantage of having a simple singular fluidic path and therefore the potential for better biocompatibility. In this configuration the magnetic bearings may be used to stabilize the axial and radial linear displacement of the rotor.

Centrifugal blood pumps, such as the Levacor [28], MitiHeart [29, 30], and Duraheart [31, 32], commonly also use actuators that act through the "back clearance" or the typically bladeless area underneath the impeller and above the stator. In this orientation, the actuators are exerting a force over a fairly large flat area and the magnetic gap is perpendicular to the axis of rotation. In some centrifugal pumps, actuators are placed along the outer diameter of the impeller or even within the spindle of the lower housing that protrudes up and through the impeller.

2.6.2 Hydrodynamically assisted suspension

It is possible to support most degrees of freedom using passive magnetic bearings and the remaining DOF using a hydrodynamic bearing. This strategy is the basis for mVAD [27] and HVAD [33]. All hydrodynamic bearings, whether radial or axial, require that the rotor be spinning, so these systems are not levitated when the rotor is static and require at least some brief period of start-up during which hydrodynamic forces increase as a function of rotational speed, but are initially not strong enough to keep the rotor from rubbing against the stator. Once the system reaches adequate rotational speed, the pump can run at steady state while completely suspended. Blood pumps are well suited to this strategy in that once the pump is initially started in clinical use there is no need to frequently, if ever, stop and then restart the pump. The tribological properties of blood, in combination with careful geometrical design of the pump's fluidic components, can be used to suspend an impeller [9, 10] (see also Chapter in this issue on Mechanical Bearings). This configuration has relatively simpler magnetic components, but is subject to more complex fluidic paths. Careful design may reduce the possibility of cell damage as blood flows through the pump without compromising bearing performance, i.e., impeller stability.

2.6.3 Motor assisted suspension

It is also possible to actively control the position of the impeller by using the existing stator coils and rotor motor components to exert electromechanical forces. This configuration is called a self-bearing motor [34, 35]. Individual motor windings always exert a radial force on the rotor, but in a typical motor, these are energized symmetrically so as to exert a zero net force on the rotor. In the typical six-pole motor, for example, opposed poles are energized simultaneously so that the resultant force may exert a torque about the rotational axis, but does not exert any net translational force because the poles are acting opposite one another. If the fluxes through these opposed pairs were not equivalent, the pair would exert both a rotational torque and a translations force on the impeller, thereby creating a combined motor/bearing. This controlled force may be accomplished by a second set of coils; each stator leg has a motor coil and a bearing coil. This strategy allows for opposed bearing coils and opposed pairs of motor coils to be connected to one another, as they would be in a typical component and to be driven by standard motor or bearing controllers. This combination of motor and bearing function may also be accomplished by combining the motor commutation effort and bearing effort into one control law (aka control algorithm) so that a single coil is used on each pole, but the current delivered to that pole is controlled independently, via separate cabling, of the opposed pole.

3 Position sensors

In order for the bearing controller to determine what force should be exerted onto the rotor, the position of the rotor must be measured. This mechanism of measuring the position of the rotor is used as *feedback* to the control law and is generally independent of the actuators described above. This section describes some of the more common methods of position measurement used in magnetic bearing systems. In general, they are all non-contacting, as a position sensor that had to physically touch the rotor would eliminate most of the advantages of using magnetic bearings for suspension. As was the case with actuators, blood pumps have the additional complication of requiring at least some amount of blood to be between the rotor and the stator, which makes the implementation of many methods of position measurement impractical.

3.1 Eddy current sensors

Eddy currents are induced in electrically conductive material when a conductor is exposed to a time-varying magnetic field, which could be caused by either the relative motion of the field source and conductor or by variations of the source strength. The time-varying magnetic field causes a circulating flow of electrons, or current, within the body of the conductor. These flowing electrons thus induce magnetic fields. The induced currents are stronger as a function of applied magnetic field, greater electrical conductivity of the conductor, and the rate of field changes. Eddy current based position sensors take advantage of this physical effect. A high frequency alternating current runs through the air-coil embedded in a stator and will induce eddy current in the conductive objective (rotor) whose position is to be measured. Usually the excitation frequency is in the range of 1–2 MHz resulting in the bandwidth of the eddy current sensor of up to 20 KHz. Variations in the electrical conductivity or magnetic permeability of the test object, the presence of any flaws, or the air gap, will cause a change in eddy current and a corresponding change in the phase and amplitude of the measured current. In practice, everything other than the air gap can be designed to remain constant so that any variation in phase or magnitude is attributable to the air gap, which corresponds to position of the rotor. These variations can be measured using a second 'receiver' coil, or by measuring changes to the current flowing in the primary 'excitation' coil [36]. Eddy current sensors are linear and reliable and widely applied in magnetic bearing applications. Unfortunately, they are negatively affected by magnetic noise and the presence of any electrically conductive material within the air gap, which generally includes a metallic wall to separate blood from the electrical pump components. Therefore, application of eddy current sensors for measuring rotor position in magnetically levitated blood pumps is a non-trivial engineering problem.

3.2 Inductance based sensors

An inductor coil is wound around a ferromagnetic core that is driven by an oscillator and points to the rotor/ferromagnetic object. Because the rotor itself is part of the magnetic flux loop, the magnetic inductance of flux loop and electrical inductance of the coils change as a function of the distance between rotor and stator. Standard electronics can measure the electrical inductance of the coil and output a voltage, thereby creating an inductance based position sensor with an output voltage proportional to the distance between the core and the objective [37].

3.3 Hall effect sensors

A Hall effect sensor is a transducer that varies its output voltage in response to the magnetic field that it is exposed to. In the typical use for position sensing, a permanent magnet is placed within the rotor and this magnet generates a field that can be detected by a Hall effect sensor located within the stator. The air gap/distance is in the magnetic flux loop and it affects the magnetic field density and therefore the output voltage [38]. Because the magnitude of the magnetic field is a function of distance from the permanent magnet, proper design and calibration can relate the output voltage of the sensor to the position of the rotor. Hall effect sensors are fast and have wide frequency response, but can be very sensitive to magnetic noise.

3.4 Optical sensors

Reflectance-based optical sensors are commonly used to measure position. The reflectance optical sensor has a light-emitting diode focused onto the objective and the reflected light is received by a photo-diode. The intensity of reflected light varies with gap/distance between the sensor and the rotor/objective. The optical sensor will have high bandwidth and high linearity for displacement measurement, but the requirement of optical access through the biocompatible blood contacting surface and through the blood makes these difficult to implement in blood pumps.

3.5 Capacitive sensors

Capacitor displacement sensors are non-contact probes whose capacitance varies with the gap between the probe head and the target [37]. The probe head carries one electrode and the rotor/objective carries the second electrode. The voltage between the two is proportional to the gap. Capacitor displacement sensors can have very high resolution and high bandwidth for AMB position sensing application, but they are very sensitive to magnetic noise and also susceptible to static charge on the rotor/target. For maglev blood pump application, the blood properties may change the dielectric permittivity of the medium. Most importantly, these may be impossible to implement in a truly levitated system because they require electrical contact with the rotor.

3.6 Self-sensing magnetic bearings

Self-sensing bearings attempt to use a single coil and iron core as both the actuator and position sensor. In the same way that inductance based sensors take advantage of the fact that the electrical inductance varies as a function of proximity of the rotor, the inductance of the actuator itself varies as a function of rotor position, being approximately inversely proportional to the air gap distance. The measurement of inductance of a coil is complicated by having to use that same coil as an actuator, but methods to measure the inductance using signals of substantially higher frequency than the control effort have been demonstrated [39]. The main challenge remains separating dynamic information needed to control the bearings from noise and residual control signals. There are different methods for filtering coil voltages, but a common approach is to examine the range of frequencies corresponding to the mechanical dynamic range of the rotor system, because displacements are expected to occur in this interval. Further, demodulation filters are used to extract the displacement information from the coil currents.

In a blood pump, this method has the obvious advantage of reducing wires and system complexity by eliminating the need for a separate position sensor in the AMB system. The elimination of displacement sensors can also improve system reliability. Furthermore, a rotor-bearing system can be designed to be shorter and stiffer without a discrete displacement sensor that takes up some physical space (typically axial length) on the rotor. In addition, the problem of sensor/actuator non-collocation, which may cause system instability, can be resolved. Lastly, if the method of self-sensing parameter estimation is used, the need for noise filtering circuits is eliminated because the Pulse Width Modulation (PWM) switching signal is used as information on displacement rather than as noise.

4　Controller and electronics design

The controller is critical to the function and performance of the active magnetic bearing (AMB) and therefore, the entire levitation system, as shown in Figure 4. The controller includes the hardware and software that interprets the measurement of position of the impeller and determines what force each actuator should exert. Within this section, we describe the fundamental elements of a controller, and one of the most common control strategies typically employed to achieve rotor stability are proportional-integral-derivative (PID). The remainder of the section includes a brief description of more advanced control scheme and of some of the hardware elements typical to a controller.

4.1　Design principle of one-axis suspension

The linearized force/current and force/displacement relationship of electromagnets at the operating point (equilibrium position: i_0, s_0) was expressed in Equation 2, but is repeated here for reference:

$$F(i, s)_d = \kappa_d i_d - K_d s_d \qquad d = x, y, z \tag{3}$$

κ_d is the current stiffness of the actuator in the d direction. Since active magnetic bearings have a negative passive bearing stiffness, K, in the controlled coordinate direction, the magnetic bearings are open loop unstable. The control system has to provide the restoring force and damping force to overcome the negative bearings stiffness via the control current, like the typical second order mass-spring-damper system. This corresponding force with stiffness K and damping δ can be expressed as:

$$f = -Ks - \delta \dot{s} \tag{4}$$

4.2　Control laws

Given an actuator that can exert force to move the rotor and a means of sensing position of the rotor, a control scheme needs to have some way of determining how strong and in which direction to exert force. The study and design of control laws is certainly not limited to magnetic bearings, and applies to essentially any system where controlled variable is modulated in order to achieve a desired system response. This could include modulation of your furnace for control of house temperature, modulation of an airfoil orientation for control of an aircraft, or modulation of force generated by an active magnetic bearing for control of position of a blood pump impeller. Although it is not covered in this chapter, but should be noted that control theory is also applied to motor speed for regulating blood flow, or to physiological loads and prevention of side effects (such as right ventricular failure) [40–44] within the field of blood pumps.

Most typically, the effect of the controller variable and the response of the system are modeled according to a set of mathematical equations, referred to as state. This section focuses on the control laws used to achieve rotor suspension through a generalized relationship between the actuator forces discussed in the previous section, i.e., $f = f(i, s) \leftrightarrow f_k(i_k, x_k)$, and a set of k state variables, x_k, observed with different sensors discussed in Chapter 3 and modulated with control currents, i_k. For simplicity, we assume there is one actuator per sensor, but that need not be the case. A block diagram illustrating the basic signals and systems of a magnetic bearing control system is shown in Figure 12.

The concept of stability is central to the design of a control law. The formal mathematical definition can be found elsewhere [45, 46], but in magnetically suspended bearing systems, it can be intuitively derived as

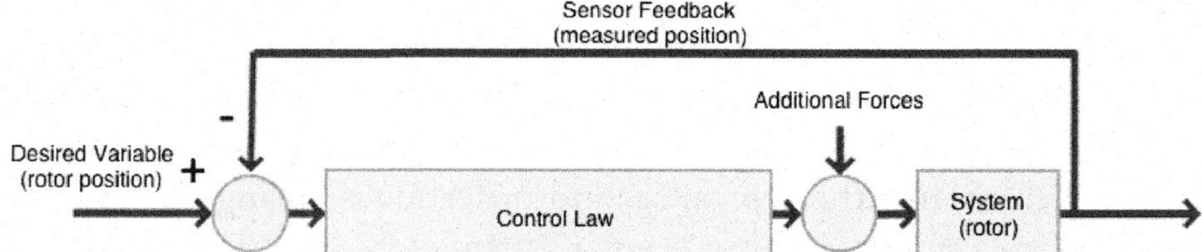

Figure 12 The magnetic bearings in an assist device are generally designed to keep the rotor magnetically suspended within a desired distance from the housing. A negative-feedback control law uses the distance between the desired and actual position to calculate a control force. Ultimately, the bearing system responds to the control force as well as external influences, which could include gravity and hydrodynamic forces. The rotor moves in response to these forces, depending on the properties of the system, which would account for the inertia and rotation of the impeller, and the new position is measured by the sensors in the system.

the need for an additional *active* force arising from the fundamental inability to fully suspend a rotor by *passive* magnets described in Section 1.1.1.

Another useful concept in the development and implementation of control laws consists of mathematical transforms, primarily the Laplace transform, which enables simplification of temporal signals, differential and integral relationships, stability criteria, and input/output relationships through transfer functions [45, 46]. Transfer functions allow compartmentalization of systems involved in the control of the assist device. Subsystems and signals can be sequentially incorporated by means of transfer functions in the Laplace domain, i.e., where the complex variable, s, is the independent variable.

4.2.1 Proportional, integral, and derivative (PID)

Proportional Integral Derivative (PID) control is one of the most common control laws and is generally successful in magnetic bearing applications. This control law consists of the summation of proportional, integral, and derivative components and each of these is described here. Perhaps the simplest control law consists of applying a force in the opposite direction to the rotor displacement from its desired position, i.e., if the rotor is to the right of its target position then push to the left. If this force is a function of how far the location is from desired position, this is known as *proportional control*, i.e., if the rotor is further to the right then push harder to the left.

It is often useful to the controller to use information about the velocity in addition to position information. For example, imagine that the impeller is quickly moving from left to right, but just passing the desired position at this instant in time. It may make sense to push to the left, even though the instantaneous location is fine. At this instant, proportional control would yield no control effort, but *derivative control*, would result in a control effort. In this example, velocity is the first temporal derivative of our controlled variable, position.

It can be shown that a control law typically needs at least PD control to maintain stability [47]. If only proportional and derivative control, a PD control law, it is common that a stable state is reached, but that this state is not the exact desired state. If any steady external force is acting, such as gravity acting on the rotor in our example, then some distance between the desired and actual state exists at steady state so that there is a control effort from the proportional term to counteract the external force. In order to overcome this problem, *integral control* is used. The integrator acts to bring this steady and stable position back to the desired position by adding a control effort that is a function of the integral of the error. When the position error in the control loop has decreased to zero, the integrator state remains unchanged, and the system reaches stability and the zero offset position.

Proportional Integral Derivative (PID) control, the most common control laws in magnetic bearing applications, simply sums these three terms (Equation 5). Here x_k indicates the error, or the position as compared to the desired position. The P, I, and D terms appear in order on the right hand side of the equation. Each term has a coefficient, or *gain*, c, that could be used to adjust the relative magnitude of each term. Notice that a negative actuator force, f_k, results from a positive position error, a positive integral of error, or a positive velocity.

$$f_k = -\left(c_p x_k + c_i \int x_k dt + c_d \frac{dx_k}{dt} \right) \tag{5}$$

The design of a PID control laws consists of setting appropriate gains for each degree of freedom of the system. This can be done from theory or numerical modeling using an accurate model of the sensors, actuators, and system dynamics. Although PID control is versatile and relatively accessible in terms of practical implementation, it is susceptible to controller-induced instability, which occurs when a particular set of feedback coefficients result in the generation of control forces that actually disturb and destabilize the system (e.g., increased derivative gain may actually amplify noise). To avoid controller-induced instability the controller must be manually tuned to perform in a variety of situations, or augmented by advanced control algorithms.

4.2.2   Advanced control laws

The design of control laws is an entire field of engineering. Although all control laws share the same basic goal, reducing the error of a measured variable by exerting some control effort, numerous methods have been presented, analyzed and employed. Most typically, these are aimed at dealing with uncertainty or variability in the sensors or the model of the system. Some of these advanced control laws are described at the most elementary level here, and some references are included for further reading.

Virtual Zero Power (VZP) control has been used in magnetic suspension systems with permanent magnets providing bias flux. This control realizes the steady states in which the coil current converges to zero with time and the force produced by the permanent magnets balances the weight of the suspended object. In effect, it replaces the force from the integral term of the PID controller with the first term of Equation 3, which is a force due to the relative alignment of the permanent magnets. Because there is no steady energy consumption for the stable levitation, it is desired in applications like aerospace, and magnetically-levitated heart pumps where low energy consumption is strongly required [48]. It is to be noted that power supply is also needed even at steady state to continue the stabilization via active control.

Linear-Quadratic-Gaussian is a composite control strategy based on both sensor feedback and an ideal system model. Rotor dynamics are inherently nonlinear due, for the most part, to the rotational components and fluidic interaction. Nevertheless, it is possible to obtain a reasonable *linear* system model within a certain working range. In that case, it is possible to obtain a closed-form expression of feedback gains that will achieve stability with the least amount of energy. The gains are desirable because they promise optimal rotor performance and low power consumption, and arise from the minimization of a quadratic energy functional of user-defined weights (the linear quadratic regulator). However, since the optimal solution is only valid within the linear operating range, additional measures must be taken account for sensor feedback and nonlinear system performance. The so-called Kalman filter [49], or state observer, allows combination of a linear system model through a series of weights aimed at reducing the least-squares difference between the sensor output and the system model. Thus, enabling near-optimal operation in the linear range, as well as robust operation in the nonlinear range.

The basic concept of *dynamic inversion* is to use a system model to completely remove the open-loop (or uncontrolled) system dynamics and replace it by stable dynamics [45]. A simple implementation of dynamic inversion consists of two models, one for the open-loop bearing system, and another one for the closed-loop response [45]. Compared to a basic PID controller, dynamic inversion control laws are desired because it gives the designer more complete control of system response even in the presence of nonlinearities and multiple inputs or outputs. It does, however, require more computing power and accurate mathematical representation of the physical system [45].

To relieve modeling inaccuracies, *sliding mode control* uses dynamic inversion combined with a more conventional negative-feedback controller, such as PID. Sliding mode control uses a switching approach to make the system states remain on a state of dynamic inversion (sliding surface) by design of the switching strategy and control law. Properly deployed, sliding-mode control is able to sustain changes in the fundamental behavior of the system, such as those due to variations in hemodynamics or low battery power [50]. It does, however, require empirical tuning parameters to optimize controller performance [47, 51].

Adaptive Control Laws use information stored in memory to update coefficients [45]. For instance, calculating low-frequency variations in bearing force, and then using this information to update integral control coefficients can be useful to counteract preload variations on the pump due to varying heart rate. Specific applications of adaptive controllers are diverse and include adaptation to physiological response, electronic interference, and error tolerance [45, 52, 53].

The *bi-quadratic filter* is a useful control strategy for AMBs by reshaping the rotor-bearing transfer function, so that it includes second-order dynamics explicitly. A second-order representation of the controller allows a more direct assessment of stability by means of mathematical analysis (evaluating the eigenvalues of the controller's characteristic equation). This analytical flexibility is especially useful with deformable rotors, which not only respond to forces as a rigid object, but also include spring-like behaviors such as bending.

Lead-lag compensation is a classical method included in more advanced control laws in order to reshape the frequency response of the system and thus improve the overall system response.

4.3 Hardware

The hardware components used for magnetic bearing applications depend on the type of magnetic bearing (active, passive, hybrid), and design-specific characteristics (degrees of freedom, speed range). For magnetic bearings that require some kind of active control, the hardware is identical to many other control applications, but with the reliability requirements for medical assist devices. A generalized digital control system consists of three basic components: (1) Analog to Digital Converters (ADC, or A/D converters), which digitize analog input signals from position sensors, a (2) Processor, which calculates the forces and torques needed to control the bearing system, and (3) Digital to Analog Converters (DAC, or D/A converters), which convert a digital signal into an analog actuation signal. In addition to these components, additional signal conditioning elements such as filters and amplifiers are used to reduce sensor noise and create the power required for actuation. Contemporary components may integrate these. For example, digital control applications use A/D converters with built-in antialiasing filters and some power amplifiers may perform D/A conversion.

While early industrial AMB control implementations in the 1970s and 80s were realized in analog electronics, digital control has taken over for the majority of applications since the early 1990s due to progress in microprocessor and peripheral device technology. Examples include the appearance of fast signal processors, analog-to-digital (A/D) and digital-to-analog (D/A) converter as well as pulse width modulation (PWM) units.

4.3.1 Analog-to-digital conversion and data acquisition

The output of many sensors is an analog voltage that has to be converted to a digital signal for the controller to operate on this information. As is the case for most electronics, analog to digital conversion (A/D) is becoming less expensive each year. These are typically sized by the speed requirements (samples per second) and the accuracy of the digitization of the signal; 12 or 14 bit converters are common. Historically, these could be purchased as discrete units, but are now commonly incorporated into micro-processors to form a micro-controller.

4.3.2 Processor

As an example, the Texas Instrument C28X core is a current (2014) example of a high performance DSP core for digital control applications. The 32-bit F2812 has on board 256KB flash, 36KB RAM, 16 channels 12 bits ADC and runs at 150MHz, making it capable of numerous sophisticated control algorithms in real-time including magnetic bearings control, sensorless motor speed control, random PWM and power factor correction. AMB designers and manufacturers have benefited from the enhanced flexibility, durability and added capabilities of digital control. Newer processors have benefits to the end user and product quality because built-in instrumentation in conjunction with digital control can offer a host of insights into machine internal quantities, such as process forces or balancing quality, which would not be as readily accessible with other bearing technologies. Moreover, thanks to the various interfacing capabilities of a modern digital AMB control system, the end-user can easily integrate it into an overall machine control system.

4.3.3 Power amplifier

There are two types of power amplifiers: linear amplifiers and switching amplifiers. Linear amplifiers are usually easy to operate, signals are clean and there is little disturbance from the noise, but the heat loss is very large; a small amount of power is delivered to the actuator coil and the remainder is converted to waste heat. Switching amplifiers have a very high power efficiency compared to linear amplifiers, but the switching creates electrical noise, and may affect the signals of position sensors.

5 Performance considerations of magnetic bearings in VADs

In the US, device failure still accounts for approximately 8% of re-admittance of patients being treated for left-ventricular dysfunction using VADs [54]. Though magnetic bearings offer a viable solution to extend design life of pumps and to reduce shear stress and heat generation associated with mechanical bearings, they do introduce an additional suite of complications. In many aspects, such as evaluating the theoretical reduction of thromboembolic potential when using wide-gap magnetic bearing configurations, the facts are obscured by challenges associated with assessing the true performance of devices in controlled environments, such as numerical simulations, bench-top experiments, or animal testing. Further, data from human trials in a large enough sample size requires years to obtain, and is seldom equivalent to a controlled environment. Nevertheless, pumps using magnetic suspension have to perform comparably to existing mechanical bearing devices in the short-term for them to be preferred by physicians and patients. The basic considerations necessary to achieve comparative performance, some of them unique to magnetic bearings, include size, battery life, ease and reliability of connectors, and the cable stiffness and diameter, some of which are discussed in this chapter.

5.1 System complexity

The inclusion of a magnetic bearing system necessarily means more components in the system. This includes additional wires to supply current to the actuators and to transmit the position sensor output to the controller. While it is plausible that the sensor signal may be transmitted through a very low capacity wire or wirelessly in the future, the power to the bearings is substantial enough that these wires are typically of a gage similar to the motor windings. A typical mechanical bearing pump, such as the HeartMate II may use as few as three wires (six in order to maintain full redundancy) to supply the brushless DC motor. Magnetic bearing devices contain at least an additional four for a single degree of active control and some pumps contain many more total wires. This increases the size of the so-called "drive-line" and required connectors, both at the external controller and to the pump. Magnetic bearing pumps are also outfitted with active components, such as sensors and other electronics. Although electronic components follow the same reliability trends that have encouraged replacement of moving parts with solid-state technology in other technologies, they do increase the overall complexity of the system and require special manufacturing and care considerations. The application of digital systems and the possibility of wireless connectivity has made, compatibility and security areas of concern.

5.2 Weight and size

In order to be accepted by the medical community the pump must be able to fit within the torso in a manner similar to existing pumps. One limitation of magnetic bearing systems is that they have a fairly large volume as compared to a mechanical bearing system. The inclusion of additional components related to the magnetic bearing system increases the size of the pump as compared to an analogous design that uses mechanical bearings. This is reflected in the trends of miniaturization during the past ten years. Recent pumps using mechanical bearings, such as the Jarvik 2000 (29cc) and MicroMed (50cc) are only a fraction of the size of the HeartMate II (112cc), whereas state-of-the-art magnetically levitated blood pumps are of similar size or even larger (82cc INCOR, 150cc Levacor). Hydrodynamic assisted suspensions address this by eliminating the need for active bearings (hVAD 50cc and mVAD apparently <15cc).

5.3 Power consumption

Power delivered to a pump is transferred, via the motor and impeller, to the fluid. In most pumps, a part of the incoming usable energy is added to the fluid and some is lost to bearing friction. Nonetheless, mechanical bearings themselves do not use a lot of energy, so that the net power saved by reducing friction with the usage of magnetic bearings is negligible. In fact, the power consumed by a magnetically suspended pump is higher than a well-designed mechanically suspended pump, because the active magnetic bearings will require additional energy input. Because passive components of the system do not consume power, some hybrid (active/passive) magnetic bearings designs use passive components for relatively heavy loads so that active components use less energy. Similarly, some pumps with active control in the main load bearing direction, such as the axial suspension in the Levacor, make use of low-power-consumption control algorithms. Particular pump designs are discussed in more detail in a later section of this chapter. Having said this, most of the magnetically suspended pumps designed in the era of computational fluid dynamics, have excellent flow paths and relatively high hydraulic efficiency leading to net power consumption similar, or better, than their predecessors. Some examples of power requirements include the MitiHeart, which consumes 6W for rotation and <0.5W for the magnetic suspension [55], and the INCOR, which reports a total power use less than 4W [56].

Although there is evidence that the presence of the blood within the magnetic flux path does not interfere with the bearing performance, there are additional material selection constraints imposed on devices that use magnetic bearings that are not present in a mechanical bearing system. In particular, the magnetic permeability of the material between the rotor and stator must be low enough to not interfere with the magnetic flux passing between the rotor and the stator and the electrical conductivity must be adequately low to minimize interference from eddy currents.

5.4 Physical disturbance rejection

The implanted pump can experience many different types of physical disturbances to the stator. These range from those experienced during typical daily life (walking, climbing stairs) to exercise conditions. Accelerations of the torso have been shown to be as high as 10 times the force of gravity for typical running. More extreme conditions may be experienced during traumatic events, such as falling, an automobile accident or the torso being struck by an object. Most magnetic bearing pumps are designed so that typical loads due to walking and running will not cause part of the bearing to momentarily collide with another surface or "touch down". A short duration high force disturbance may cause the bearing to instantaneously touch the wall, so the bearing must be designed so that the rotor suspension immediately resumes after an event, so that the motor continues to run. There is a trade-off between physical disturbance rejection and power consumption, so that more robust systems will generally require more power. Although control algorithms can be updated with relative ease given an existing system, decisions regarding the level of robustness of a device need to be considered during the design phase because they can affect many components and alter their performance. For instance the frequency response and noise level of the sensors, force capacity of the actuators, and the form or tuning parameters of the control law affects stability.

5.5 Reliability and durability

In general, reliability is the ability of a system to perform and maintain function in routine as well as hostile or unexpected circumstances. Durability is the ability to perform this function over an extended period of time. In order to increase the reliability and durability of magnetic bearings systems and reduce the probability of system failures, designers incorporate redundancy, condition monitoring and alarms, and fault tolerance both in software and hardware. These may take the form of auxiliary bearings, robust control, and smart machines technologies.

All implantable blood pumps must be designed to operate for the design life without any maintenance. This makes this technology fairly unique, even among turbomachines (i.e., jet engines, gas compressors, hydro turbines), which typically allow for and require scheduled maintenance if they are to provide many years of service. Most mechanical bearings are rated to a certain duration that is a function of the hours of operation, load, and speed. Magnetic bearings, however, have no moving parts to maintain so long as they are functioning properly. It is because of the lack of moving parts subject to fatigue and mechanical wear that magnetically levitated pumps show the promise of lasting many years. As there are no moving parts, the failure modes are not mechanical, such as those that have plagued pulsatile pumps with flexing diaphragms and prosthetic valves. Nonetheless, all machines are subject to failure and the following sections discuss some of the issues with reliability within magnetically suspended blood pumps. Reliability and durability are critical with blood pumps, as is the case for all Class III devices according to the U.S. Food Drug Administration (CFR Title 21, ch. 1, part 870).

5.5.1 Sensor failure

Position sensing is a fundamental part of active magnetic bearing control so, total position sensor failure may result not only on loss of stability, but also to actuator overload due to control feedback. Given the relatively large amount of current necessary to achieve robust rotor control, failure-driven actuator overload may cause overheating. Partial sensor failure, for example a bias voltage or miscalibration, may not necessarily result in rotor instability, but can affect speed or pressure estimations, providing erroneous performance assessment. Some pumps are being developed with redundant position sensors and fault detection and or tolerance schemes built into the controller. Ideally, if any single position sensor fails, the control law can determine which sensor is failed and then still determine the states of the rotor and continue active control. Also, given proper protection from liquids to avoid possible shorts, sensor failure is less likely to occur compared to components more exposed to mechanical fatigue like wires and connectors.

5.5.2 Wire and coil failure

If an actuator coil or wires supplying current to the coils is broken, this interrupts the current path and that actuator will cease to function. Segments of wires can be damaged by excessive electrical current, which leads to joule heating, or repeated mechanical bending, which can lead to fatigue failure of the wires. Protection of circuits by software controls and physical fusing is very standard in all power electronics, so the damage from excessive current is unlikely.

Fatigue failure from mechanical bending is a much more difficult problem because of the long durations that the pump must survive and the circuitous and dynamic path that the pump driveline must take between the external controller and the implanted pump. Stress is created in every wire at locations that the cable is bent and movement of the patient's body can lead to repeated bending and unbending of the driveline, which may eventually lead to failure. Stress concentrations and sudden bends often occur within the cable just near a rigid connection or constraint of the cable and this has led to some complications with device drive lines near the external controller. The natural breathing and cardiac cycle may induce small movement to the pump and cable and common motions, such as sitting and standing, can introduce extreme movements to the cable. To further complicate matters, some patients "twiddle" the driveline, introducing tight bends. The business of strain relieving cables is as old as cabling itself, but this application represents an extreme demands as engineers are pushed to decrease wire gages to maintain a small-diameter and flexible percutaneous cable that is still viable for many years.

5.5.3 Controller durability

Because the magnetically levitated blood pumps have no moving mechanical parts, the predominant failure mechanisms are associated with electronics, rather than mechanical failures. Many failures with the 2nd generation rotary pumps have been associated with controller electronics or cables. Cable failures were addressed above and the controller's durability is determined by the durability of the controller box, circuit board, and electrical components. For mechanical durability, the temperature test and vibration test are usually needed to determine the temperature and vibration limit of the controller. In general, solid-state devices operate very reliably for long periods of time so long as they are used within their nominal ranges of operation.

5.6 Failure remediating measures

5.6.1 Manufacturing

In order to maintain the durability of electrical components, there is usually a current limit setting implemented both in software and hardware to increase the controller's durability. In order to reduce the failure of the assembly, some standards in electronics manufacturing can be followed. These include: (1) Solder paste alloy selection (traditional 63Sn/37Pb Wt% or Pb-free), (2) Component sourcing and alloy availability (some components are only available in Pb-free alloys, which can result in mixed alloy assembly and reliability concerns), (3) Under fill to ruggedize the solder joints of area array components; and (4) use of conformal coating to provide environmental protection.

5.6.2 Physical redundancy of components sensors and wires

Redundancy is one of the simplest and most effective remediating measures. Physical redundancy of wires, for example is implemented simply by having two wires in parallel. Because current will seek the path of least resistance, the fracture of one of these wires will have almost no effect on operation of the device. In most pumps, full redundancy is used within the driveline for all critical signals, including position measurements and power to the motor and actuators.

5.6.3 Fault tolerant control

Fault detection and tolerance to sensor failure may be added using software. In AMB suspension control, the fault tolerant feature is added to switch modes of operation automatically following the detection of position sensor fault. One strategy, viable when redundant sensors are available, is to reroute sensor outputs, effectively ignoring the faulty sensor, so that the main dynamic control law continues to operate. Likewise, self-sensing magnetic bearings can be used in conjunction to position sensors to achieve redundancy. In this case, the routing may include filtering or dynamic conditioning so that one sensing scheme can be used instead of another. Lastly, it is possible to switch to a mode of operation where the main dynamic control law is altogether changed for one specifically designed to perform in particular failure modes, for instance in conjunction with the auxiliary means of rotor stability.

5.6.4 Touch-down bearings

The best way to build a safe system is to make it fail-safe. In general, fail-safe means that if any component fails, the system will resort to a safe, although not nominal condition. Some AMB systems are equipped with auxiliary bearings or touch-down bearings, in order to achieve a fail-safe system. In the context of circulatory assist devices, touch-down bearings are an additional set of active or passive bearings, designed to provide rotor stability when the contact-free suspension provided by the AMB fails. Touchdown bearings may also share the transient or continuous rotor overload with magnetic bearings taking the entire load when magnetic bearings fail. Due to its association with impact and contact mechanics, the dynamics of rotor touchdown and device operation on the auxiliary bearings are very complex and non-linear. For high speed heavy machines, the life of touch-down bearings may be only about 4 coast downs [57]; in contrast, some blood pumps are able to continue spinning and running for long periods of time so that they patient may be able to have a pump replacement. Tough intricate active touchdown configurations exist [57], but passive touchdown bearings are usually simple retainer or special ball bearings. In pumps, these are typically incorporated into the design of inducer, impeller, or diffuser blades so that the impeller will touch at a desired spot. Alternatively, auxiliary stability mechanisms can be achieved when some components are designed to serve as hydrodynamic bearings in the event of a failure [57–59].

6 Specific device examples

The implementation of a full magnetic suspension into a blood pump can take various forms and both centrifugal [60] and axial pumps [58] have been designed and prototyped since the mid to late 1990s. This section is meant to give a brief description of the range of devices that have gone through at least chronic animal studies. It is not meant to be exhaustive and there are still many groups working on magnetically levitated pumps that are not as far along in development and testing.

6.1 Berlin Heart INCOR

The Berlin Heart INCOR is a fully magnetically suspended axial-flow pump. Magnetic suspension is achieved using hybrid bearings placed at each end of rotor that passively constrain radial movement and actively control axial movement of the impeller. These force-exerting elements act on the axial faces of the impeller and consist of permeable material housed within the stationary inducer and diffuser of the pump, bearing coils within the pump stator, and a target material within the rotor. This pump is approximately 30mm × 120mm and weighs 200g [59]. This device is not available in the United States, but has been implanted in more than 500 people worldwide after achieving the European Conformity

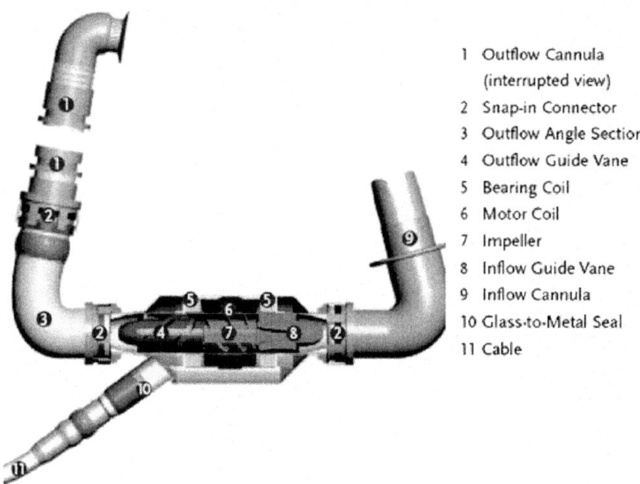

Figure 13 View of the internal components of Berlin Heart's INCOR. From http://www.berlinheart.com/englisch /medpro/incor/Pumpe/.

(CE) mark approval in 2003. The amount of force required by the magnetic bearing to suspend the rotor is a function of the pressure rise across the pump, but the manufacturer reports a very low power consumption of 3–4 W at physiological flow conditions [7].

6.2 Terumo Duraheart

The Terumo Duraheart is a fully magnetically levitated centrifugal flow pump. The magnetic bearing system actively controls the radial degrees of freedom, while supporting axial and rotational degrees of freedom passively [61, 62]. This pump is fairly large, relative to more recent pumps, measuring 65mm in diameter and 40mm in height (excluding cannulae). It has been used clinically quite extensively, first in Asia and more recently in Europe [63] and the U.S. This pump was the first to obtain the market approval (CE-mark) [64]. The magnetic

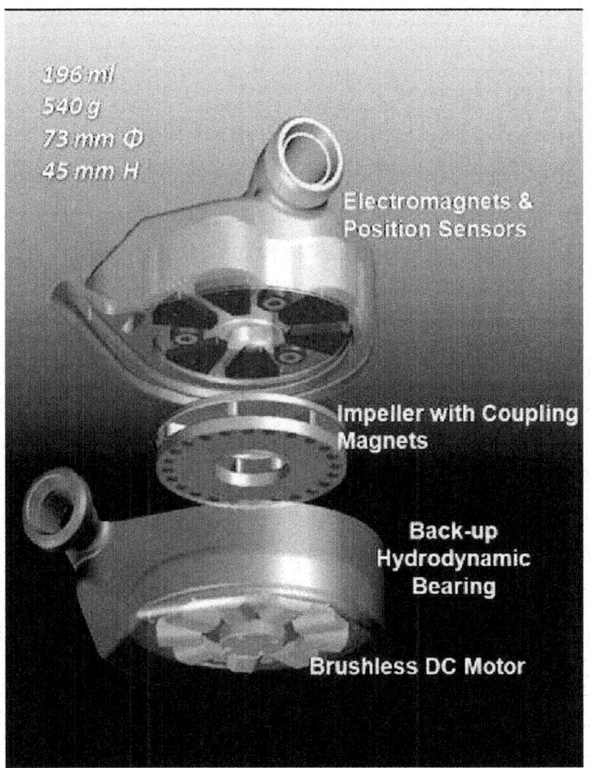

Figure 14 Exploded view of the Terumo DuraHeart. From Morshuis (2010).

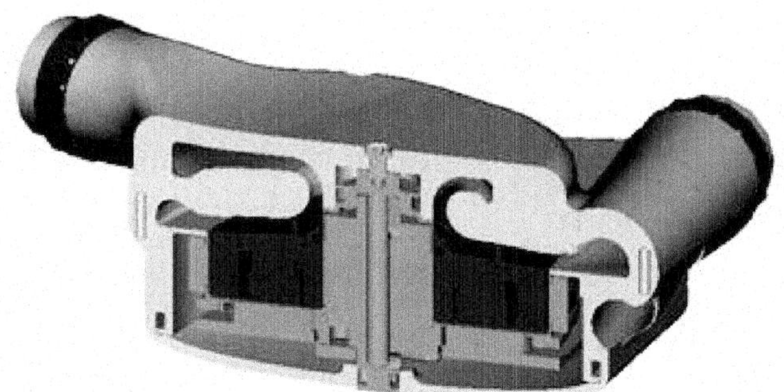

Figure 15 Sectioned view of the WorldHeart Levacor http://www.worldheart.com/index.cfm.

configuration is straightforward with position sensors and actuators in the upper portion of the stator, acting through the "front gap" onto the rotor and the motor contained within the lower portion of the stator.

6.3 WorldHeart Levacor

The Levacor pump was developed as the HeartQuest pump [17] and then became the Levacor when purchased by WorldHeart. This is a centrifugal pump with a full magnetic levitation. The radial and torsional degrees of freedom are passive and consist of permanent magnet elements within the lower stator and only the axial position of the impeller is actively controlled [65]. This single degree of freedom is actuated by a voice coil, also known as a Lorentz actuator [25, 66], located within the fixed spindle of the pump stator housing. This type of actuator is similar to the actuator on a typical audio speaker cone. There are substantial axial loads exerted onto any axial or centrifugal pump, and advanced control algorithms, such as VZP (virtually zero power) have been implemented into this suspension in order to reduce the power consumed by the magnetic bearings. This pump was used in a clinical trial in Europe, but abandoned in 2011 [59]. In this pump, permanent magnets are located within the lower stator.

6.4 PediaFlow

The PediaFlow pump is fully levitated axial-flow pump designed for use in infants and small children. In terms of suspension of the pump, there is a lot in common with the Levacor pump, in that the radial

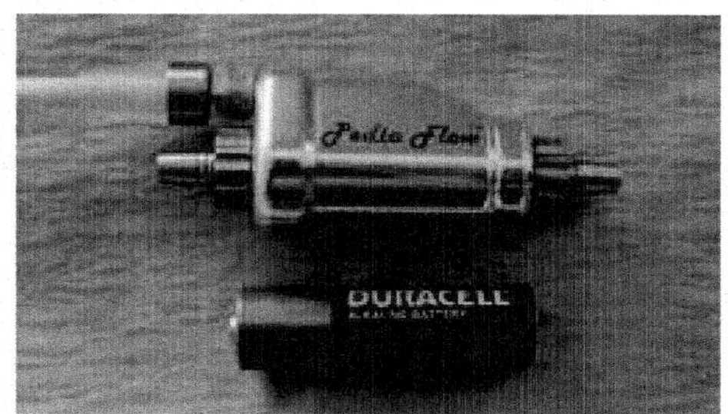

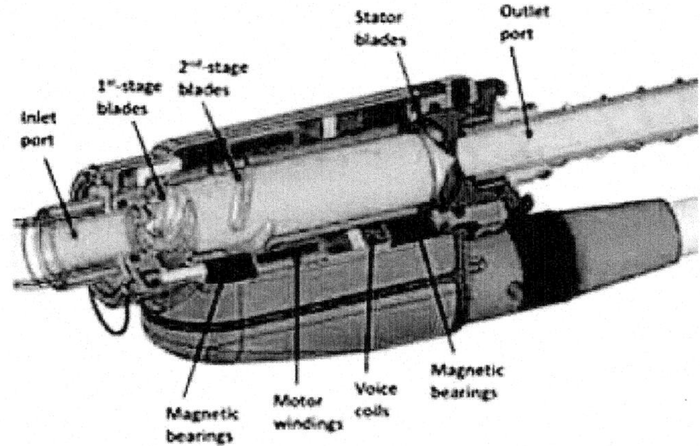

Figure 16 Exploded Pic of PediaFlow. From: http://www. launchpnt.com/portfolio/biomedical/pediaflow-pediatric-vad/.

suspension is passive and the only actively controlled degree of freedom is the axial direction [25]. In fact, because many people on the engineering team were part of the Levacor project. In fact, the magnetic suspensions are similar enough that as of 2010 or so, both pumps used the same controller hardware. The PediaFlow pump has been studied extensively [67] and is used as an example of a rigorous iterative design process including numerical models, benchtop validation prior to animal trials.

6.5 WorldHeart MiFlow VAD

This pump uses suspension and technologies as the PediaFlow, but is intended for adult usage in a small package that may be placed within the left ventricle, as is done with the mechanically supported Jarvik 2000. The MiFlow is still in development, with the company originally anticipating clinical trials by 2013 (http://www.worldheart.com/miflow. cfm). In March 2012, WorldHeart announced a definitive merger with

HeartWare, the developer of similar pumps described in the following paragraph.

6.6   Heartware HVAD and mVAD

At least one pump, the HeartWare, has adopted the strategy of using a magnetic suspension to maintain radial degrees of freedom and a hydro-dynamic bearing to support the remaining degree of freedom, the axial position. In this pump, the rotor is magnetically "stuck" to the bottom of the stator when the rotor is not spinning. The bottom surface of the impeller is designed as a hydrodynamic bearing, which slightly angled pads so that rotation creates enough axial lift to keep the impeller off of the surface. The designers have invested a considerable amount of effort into designing this surface so that it generates enough force while keeping shear stresses acceptably low. An obvious advantage of the combined passive magnetic and hydrodynamic bearing is that it requires no control algorithm to power to electromagnetic actuators.

Heartware is currently developing a new pump, the mVAD, which is a small axial-flow pump that uses a similar hybrid strategy. In this pump, the axial location is controlled by a passive magnetic repulsive bearing created by the interaction of a axially polarized ring magnet

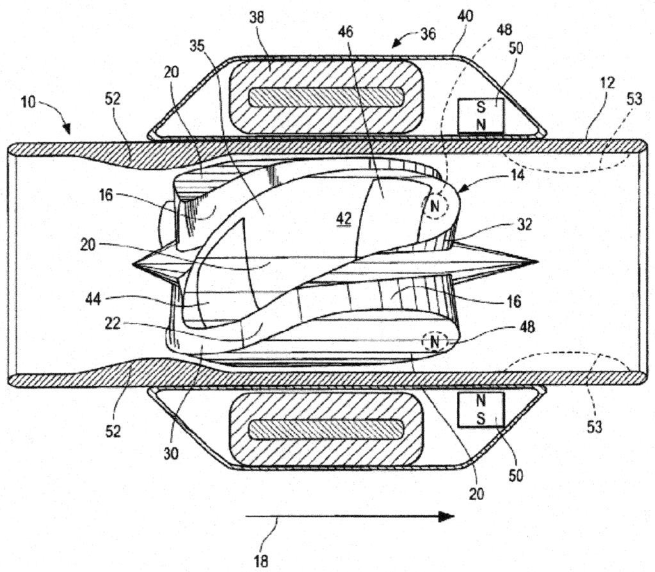

Figure 17   Sectioned view of the mVAD by HeartWare. From US Patent 7699586.

and magnets placed within each blade of the rotor. The radial restoring force is generated with wide blades with tips shaped so that the impeller blade tips form a radially stable hydrodynamic bearing when rotating.

6.7 LEV-VAD

The LEV-VAD is in a similar stage of development as the Miti Heart, having undergone animal testing, but not clinical trials. The rotor of the blood pump is supported by two identical and symmetrical hybrid magnetic bearings, each located at one end of the rotor. Unlike other pumps, these bearings are actively controlled in the radial direction and passively in the axial direction. Hall Effect Sensor Arrays (HESAs) are used to sense and deliver the radial displacements of the rotor to the HMB controller for processing. Within each HMB, a bias-flux is provided by permanent magnets (PMs) in order to decrease the system power consumption. An obvious disadvantage of having the radial direction of force be actively controlled is the need for more wires because this includes several degrees of freedom. Within this particular pump, this has actually been used to provide fault tolerant behavior, where the pump can maintain operating after any single position sensor malfunctions. An additional advantage of having the axial direction remain passive is that the highest forces exerted onto the rotor, which occur in the axial direction, are counteracted by passive elements, thereby requiring no energy. Similarly to the InCOR, the pressure rise across the pump moves the suspended impeller axially.

6.8 MitiHeart

As is the case for several of the other pumps described, permanent magnets provide passive radial support and electromagnets maintain axial stability of the rotor [29, 30]. There are two hybrid magnetic bearings, one located at each end of the rotor. In order to decrease power consumption by the bearings (reported to be <0.5W), these bearings are passively radially stable and together control only the axial location of the rotor actively. The overall topology of the pump is somewhat different from other centrifugal flow pumps in that most of the bearings sit along the outer diameter of the rotor. The structure of the magnetic bearings looks somewhat more like an axial machine with the pump impeller sitting upon the end of the rotor. The pump has undergone extensive bench-top testing demonstrating low hemolysis and recent in vivo experiments.

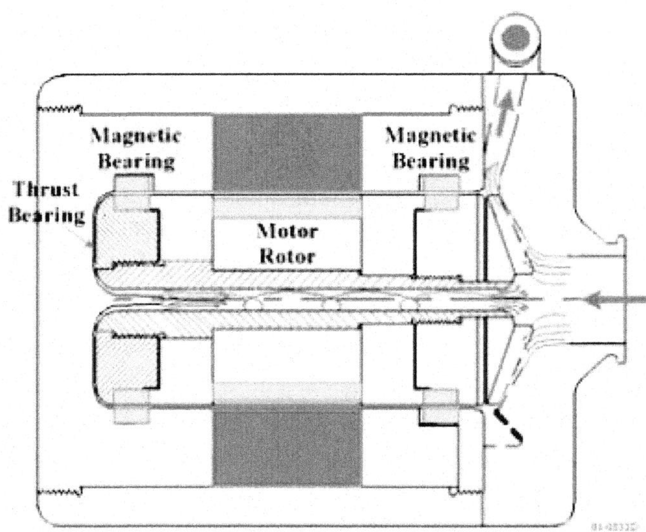

Figure 18 Cross Section of MiTiHeart showing blood path and approximate configuration of hybrid magnetic bearings [68].

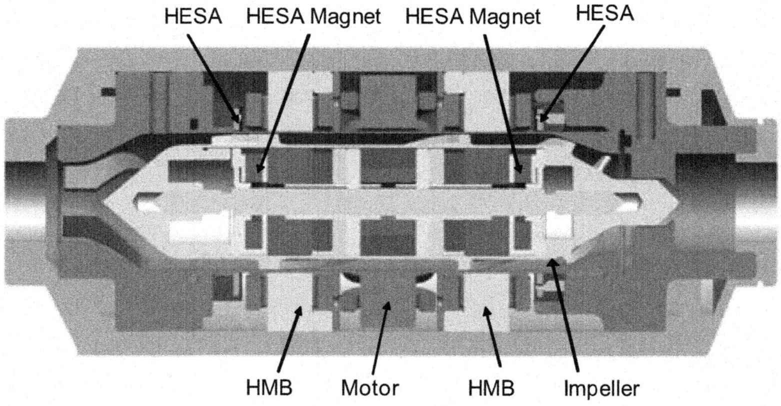

Figure 19 Longitudinal section of the LEV-VAD axial flow pump. Components of the magnetic bearing system indicated with arrows include: Hall Effect Sensor Array (HESA) and HESA magnet used for position sensing. Motor, and Hybrid Magnetic Bearing (HMB) [22].

7 Conclusion

The promise of integrating magnetic bearing systems into mechanical circulatory assist devices has been acknowledged for some time and includes patents that have since expired [69, 70]. Several decades later, many of the devices in use incorporate some aspects of magnetic bearings and a few fully magnetically suspended pumps exist, but they are still far from ubiquitous in clinical use. The most commonly implanted pumps in 2015 remain mechanically suspended rotary type devices, such as the HeartMate II. This is likely a reflection of both increased size and decreased reliability that accompany magnetic bearing system, both resulting from additional components described in this monograph. The slow adoption of this technology is also the results of the complex regulatory and scientific environment, where the true performance of mechanical assist devices is often not known until used in humans and the costs of developing a device to the point of clinical trials is enormous.

Within this chapter, we have attempted to summarize the basic design and function of a magnetic bearing system applied to a rotary mechanical assist device, aka a "blood pump". Although there are several variations of the general design of a magnetic bearing, we hope that the reader will recognize some generalities. First, permanent magnets may be arranged to generate force in a single coordinate direction using no power, but at least one active magnetic bearing must be used to completely levitate an impeller. Secondly, any active magnetic bearing requires position sensing, a control law, and electromagnetic actuator. This article does not contain enough information to allow a reader to design a magnetic bearing system, we hope that it serves as a sufficient introduction to the topic that a layperson can learn basic function and a person interested in further study can use this manuscript and included references an entry point to the their study.

8 References

[1] K. Sawada, "Outlook of the Superconducting Maglev," *Proceedings of the IEEE*, vol. 97, no. 11. pp. 1881–1885, 2009.

[2] S. Banerjee, M. K. Sarkar, P. K. Biswas, R. Bhaduri, and P. Sarkar, "A Review Note on Different Components of Simple Electromagnetic Levitation Systems," *IETE Tech. Rev.*, vol. 28, no. 3, pp. 256–264, 2011.

[3] J. A. Vazquez, E. H. Maslen, H. J. Ahn, and D. C. Han, "Model Identification of a Rotor with Magnetic Bearings," *Int. Gas Turbine Aeroengine Congr. Exhib.*, vol. 125, no. 1, p. 149, 2003.

[4] F. N. Werfel, U. Floegel-Delor, R. Rothfeld, T. Riedel, B. Goebel, D. Wippich, and P. Schirrmeister, "Superconductor Bearings, Flywheels and Transportation," *Supercond. Sci. Technol.*, vol. 25, no. 1, p. 014007, 2012.

[5] Y. Wu, C. Bingham, D. Peel, and D. Howe, "Active Magnetic Bearings for a Flywheel Peak Power Buffer for Electric Vehicles," *Internaltional Journa Appl. Electromagn. Mech.*, vol. 15, no. 1–4, pp. 201–206, 2001.

[6] D. B. Olsen, "The History of Continuous-Flow Blood Pumps," *Artif. Organs*, vol. 24, no. 6, pp. 401–404, Jun. 2000.

[7] F. D. Pagani, "Continuous-Flow Rotary Left Ventricular Assist Devices with '3rd Generation' Design," *Semin. Thorac. Cardiovasc. Surg.*, vol. 20, no. 3, pp. 255–263, Jan. 2008.

[8] C. Chen, B. Paden, J. Antaki, J. Ludlow, and G. Bearnson, "Optimal Design of Permanent Magnet Bearings with Application to the HeartQuest Ventricular Assist Device," *Jsme Int. J.*, vol. 46, no. 2, pp. 403–408, 2003.

[9] S. D. Gregory, D. Timms, N. Gaddum, D. G. Mason, and J. F. Fraser, "Biventricular Assist Devices: A Technical Review," *Ann. Biomed. Eng.*, vol. 39, no. 9, pp. 2313–2328, 2011.

[10] Y. Ando, T. Kitao, E. Nagaoka, T. Kimura, Y. Yokoyama, M. Yoshikawa, R. Tominaga, and S. Takatani, "One-Month Biocompatibility Evaluation of the Pediatric TinyPump in Goats," *Artif. Organs*, vol. 35, no. 8, pp. 813–818, 2011.

[11] L. Gentili, L. Marconi, and B. Paden, "Disturbance Rejection in the Control of a Maglev Artificial Heart," *J. Dyn. Syst. Meas. Control*, vol. 130, no. 1, p. 011003, 2008.

[12] H. Wu, Z. Wang, and X. Lv, "Design and Simulation of Axial Flow Maglev Blood Pump," *Int. J. Inf. Eng. Electron. Bus.*, vol. 3, no. 2, pp. 42–48, 2011.

[13] J. Asama, T. Shinshi, H. Hoshi, S. Takatani, and A. Shimokohbe, "A Compact Highly Efficient and Low Hemolytic Centrifugal Blood Pump with a Magnetically Levitated Impeller," *Artif. Organs*, vol. 30, no. 3, pp. 160–167, Mar. 2006.

[14] S. Yang and M. Huang, "Design and Implementation of a Magnetically Levitated Single-Axis Controlled Axial Blood Pump," *IEEE Trans. Ind. Electron.*, vol. 56, no. 6, pp. 2213–2219, Jun. 2009.

[15] M. Glauser, W. Jiang, G. Li, Z. Lin, P. E. Allaire, and D. Olson, "Optimization of an Axial Flow Heart Pump with Active and Passive Magnetic Bearings," *Artif. Organs*, vol. 30, no. 5, pp. 400–403, May 2006.

[16] T. M. Lim, S. Cheng, and L. P. Chua, "Parameter Estimation and Actuator Characteristics of Hybrid Magnetic Bearings for Axial Flow Blood Pump Applications," *Artif. Organs*, vol. 33, no. 7, pp. 509–531, 2009.

[17] P. Allaire, E. Hilton, M. Baloh, E. Maslen, G. Bearnson, D. Noh, P. Khanwilkar, and D. Olsen, " Performance of a Continuous Flow Ventricular Assist Device: Magnetic Bearing Design, Construction, and Testing." *Artif. Organs*, vol. 22, no. 6, pp. 475–490, 1998.

[18] T. Krabatsch, M. Schweiger, A. Stepanenko, T. Drews, E. Potapov, M. Pasic, Y. Weng, M. Huebler, and R. Hetzer, "Improvements in Implantable Mechanical Circulatory Support Systems. Literature Overview and Update," *Herz*, vol. 36, no. 7, pp. 622–629, 2011.

[19] S. Earnshaw, "On the Nature of the Molecular Forces which Regulate the Constitution of the Luminiferous Ether," *Trans. Cambridge Philos. Soc.*, vol. 7, pp. 97–112, 1842.

[20] B. Paden, N. Groom, and J. F. Antaki, "Design Formulas for Permanent-Magnet Bearings," *J. Mech. Des.*, vol. 125, no. 4, p. 734, 2003.

[21] F. Jiancheng, S. Jinji, X. Yanliang, and W. Xi, "A New Structure for Permanent-Magnet-Biased Axial Hybrid Magnetic Bearings," *Magn. IEEE Trans.*, vol. 45, no. 12, pp. 5319–5325, 2009.

[22] S. Cheng, M. W. Olles, A. F. Burger, and S. W. Day, "Optimization of a Hybrid Magnetic Bearing for a Magnetically Levitated Blood Pump via 3-D FEA," *Mechatronics (Oxf).*, vol. 21, no. 7, pp. 1163–1169, Oct. 2011.

[23] C. Yang, C. Knospe, P. Tsiotras, "Optimal Control of a Magnetic Bearing without Bias Flux Using Finite Voltage," Optimal Control Applications and Methods, Vol 19, Issue 4, pages 227–246, 1998.

[24] S. Cheng, M. W. Olles, A. F. Burger, and S. W. Day, "Optimization of a Hybrid Magnetic Bearing for a Magnetically Levitated Blood Pump via 3-D FEA," *Mechatronics (Oxf).*, vol. 21, no. 7, pp. 1163–1169, Oct. 2011.

[25] M. D. Noh, J. F. Antaki, M. Ricci, J. Gardiner, D. Paden, J. Wu, E. Prem, H. Borovetz, and B. E. Paden, "Magnetic Design for the PediaFlow Ventricular Assist Device," *Artif Organs*, vol. 32, no. 2, pp. 127–135, 2008.

[26] S. Cheng, M. W. Olles, D. B. Olsen, L. D. Joyce, and S. W. Day, "Miniaturization of a Magnetically Levitated Axial Flow Blood Pump," *Artif. Organs*, vol. 34, no. 10, pp. 807–815, Oct. 2010.

[27] M. S. Slaughter, M. a Sobieski, D. Tamez, T. Horrell, J. Graham, P. S. Pappas, A. J. Tatooles, and J. LaRose, "HeartWare Miniature Axial-Flow Ventricular Assist Device: Design and Initial Feasibility Test," *Tex. Heart Inst. J.*, vol. 36, no. 1, pp. 12–16, Jan. 2009.

[28] J. Bearnson, GB Jacobs, GB Kirk, J Khanwilkar, PS Nelson, KE Long, "HeartQuest Ventricular Assist Device Magnetically Levitated Centrifugal Blood Pump," *Artif. Organs*, vol. 30, no. 5, pp. 339–346, 2006.

[29] S. Jahanmir, A. Z. Hunsberger, Z. Ren, H. Heshmat, C. Heshmat, M. J. Tomaszewski, and J. F. Walton, "Design of a Small Centrifugal Blood Pump with Magnetic Bearings," *Artif Organs*, vol. 33, no. 9, pp. 714–726, 2009.

[30] Z. Ren, S. Jahanmir, H. Heshmat, A. Z. Hunsberger, and J. F. Walton, "Design Analysis and Performance Assessment of Hybrid Magnetic Bearings for a Rotary Centrifugal Blood Pump," *ASAIO J.*, vol. 55, no. 4, pp. 340–347.

[31] C. Nojiri, T. Kijima, J. Maekawa, K. Horiuchi, T. Kido, T. Sugiyama, T. Mori, N. Sugiura, T. Asada, H. Shimane, T. Ozaki, M. Suzuki, T. Akamatsu, and T. Akutsu, "Recent Progress in the Development of Terumo Implantable Left Ventricular Assist System," *ASAIO J.* vol. 45, no. 3, pp. 199–203, 1999.

[32] C. Nojiri, T. Kijima, J. Maekawa, K. Horiuchi, T. Kido, T. Sugiyama, T. Mori, N. Sugiura, T. Asada, W. Umemura, T. Ozaki, M. Suzuki, T. Akamatsu, S. Westaby, T. Katsumata, and S. Saito, "Development

Status of Terumo Implantable Left Ventricular Assist System," *Artif. Organs*, vol. 25, no. 3, pp. 237–246, 1987.

[33] E. Tuzun, K. Roberts, W. E. Cohn, M. Sargin, C. J. Gemmato, B. Radovancevic, and O. H. Frazier, "In Vivo Evaluation of the HeartWare Centrifugal Ventricular Assist Device," *Tex Hear. Inst J*, vol. 34, no. 4, pp. 406–411, 2007.

[34] Y. Okada, T. Masuzawa, K.-I. Matsuda, K. Ohmori, T. Yamane, Y. Konishi, S. Fukahori, S. Ueno, and S.-J. Kim, "Axial Type Self-Bearing Motor for Axial Flow Blood Pump," *Artif. Organs*, vol. 27, no. 10, pp. 887–891, 2003.

[35] T. M. Lim and D. Zhang, "Development of Lorentz force-Type Self-Bearing Motor for an Alternative Axial Flow Blood Pump Design," *Artif. Organs*, vol. 30, no. 5, pp. 347–353, 2006.

[36] G. Schweitzer and E. H. Maslen, *Magnetic Bearings: Theory, Design, and Application to Rotating Machinery*. Springer, 2009.

[37] D. S. Nyce, *Linear Position Sensors: Theory and Application*. John Wiley & Sons, 2004.

[38] S.-M. Yang and C.-L. Huang, "A Hall Sensor-Based Three-Dimensional Displacement Measurement System for Miniature Magnetically Levitated Rotor," *IEEE Sens. J.*, vol. 9, no. 12, pp. 1872–1878, Dec. 2009.

[39] Maslen, E. H., Montie, D. T., and Iwasaki, T., Robustness Limitations in Self-sensing Magnetic Bearings," ASME Journal of Dynamic Systems, Measurement, and Control, Vol. 128, No. 2, June 2006, pp. 197–203.

[40] J. Nienaber, M. P. Wilhelm, and M. R. Sohail, "Current concepts in the Diagnosis and Management of Left Ventricular Assist Device Infections," *Expert Rev. Anti. Infect. Ther.*, vol. 11, no. 2, pp. 201–210, Feb. 2013.

[41] Y. Wang, S. C. Koenig, M. S. Slaughter, and G. A. Giridharan, "Suction prevention and Physiologic Control of Continuous Flow Left Ventricular Assist Devices Using Intrinsic Pump Parameters," *ASAIO J.*, vol. 61, no. 2, pp. 170–177, Jan.

[42] M. Arakawa, T. Nishimura, Y. Takewa, A. Umeki, M. Ando, Y. Kishimoto, Y. Fujii, S. Kyo, H. Adachi, and E. Tatsumi, "Novel Control System to Prevent Right Ventricular Failure Induced by Rotary Blood Pump," *J. Artif. Organs*, vol. 17, no. 2, pp. 135–141, Jun. 2014.

[43] M. Vollkron, H. Schima, L. Huber, R. Benkowski, G. Morello, and G. Wieselthaler, "Development of a Suction Detection System for Axial Blood Pumps," *Artif. Organs*, vol. 28, no. 8, pp. 709–716, Aug. 2004.

[44] M. Glauser, W. Jiang, G. Li, Z. Lin, P. E. Allaire, and D. Olson, "Optimization of an Axial Flow Heart Pump with Active and Passive Magnetic Bearings," *Artif. Organs*, vol. 30, no. 5, pp. 400–403, May 2006.

[45] J. Slotine, *Applied Non-Linear Control*. Clifton: Prentice-Hall, 1991.

[46] S. Sihnners, *Control System Theory and Design*. Wiley-IEEE, 1998.

[48] M. Goldowsky, "Mini Hemoreliable Axial Flow LVAD with Magnetic Bearings—Part 2: Design description," *ASAIO J.*, vol. 48, no. 1, pp. 98–100, 2002.

[49] Kalman. *J. Basic Eng.*, vol. 82, no. 1, p. 35, Mar. 1960.

[50] M. A. Bakouri, R. F. Salamonsen, A. V Savkin, A.-H. H. Alomari, E. Lim, and N. H. Lovell, "Physiological Control of Implantable Rotary Blood Pumps for Heart Failure Patients," *Conf. Proc. ... Annu. Int. Conf. IEEE Eng. Med. Biol. Soc. IEEE Eng. Med. Biol. Soc. Annu. Conf.*, vol. 2013, pp. 675–678, Jan. 2013.

[47] A. D. Gomez, "Control of a Magnetically Levitated Ventricular Assist," MS thesis, Rochester Institute of technology, Rochester, NY, 2009.

[51] T.-J. Fu and W.-F. Xie, "A Novel Sliding-Mode Control of Induction Motor Using Space Vector Modulation Technique," *ISA Trans.*, vol. 44, no. 4, pp. 481–490, Oct. 2005.

[52] Mei-Yung Chen, Chin-Chung Wang, and Li-Chen Fu, "Adaptive Sliding Mode Controller Design of a Dual-Axis Maglev Positioning System," in *Proceedings of the 2001 American Control Conference. (Cat. No.01CH37148)*, vol. 5, pp. 3731–3736, 2001.

[53] J. D. Setiawan, R. Mukherjee, and E. H. Maslen, "Adaptive Compensation of Sensor Runout and Mass Unbalance in Magnetic Bearing Systems," in *1999 IEEE/ASME International Conference on Advanced Intelligent Mechatronics (Cat. No.99TH8399)*, pp. 800–805, 1999.

[54] P. Bonde, M. A. Dew, D. Meyer et al. National trends in readmission(REA) rates following left ventricular assist device

(LVAD) therapy. International Society for Heart and Lung Transplantation 2011 Scientific Sessions; April 14, 2011; San Diego, CA. Abstract 4.

[55] "MitiHeart Technical Specifications." [Online]. Available: http://www.mitiheart.com/#/technical-specifications/4556354199.

[56] "InCOR technical specifications." [Online]. Available: http://www.berlinheart.com/englisch/medpro/incor/Pumpe/.

[57] Gerhard Schweitzer, Eric H. Maslen, "Magnetic Bearings: Theory, Design, and Application to Rotating Machinery." Springer-Verlag, 2009.

[58] Z. J. Wu, R. K. Gottlieb, G. W. Burgreen, J. A. Holmes, D. C. Borzelleca, M. V Kameneva, B. P. Griffith, and J. F. Antaki, "Investigation of Fluid Dynamics Within a Miniature Mixed Flow Blood Pump," *Stand*, vol. 31, pp. 615–629, 2001.

[59] D. Timms, "A Review of Clinical Ventricular Assist Devices," *Med. Eng. Phys.*, vol. 33, no. 9, pp. 1041–1047, Nov. 2011.

[60] G. Bearnson, E. Maslen, and D. Olsen, "Development of a Prototype Magnetically Suspended Rotor Ventricular Assist Device," *ASAIO*, pp. 275–281, 1996.

[61] C. Nojiri, T. Kijima, J. Maekawa, K. Horiuchi, T. Kido, T. Sugiyama, T. Mori, N. Sugiura, T. Asada, W. Umemura, T. Ozaki, M. Suzuki, T. Akamatsu, S. Westaby, T. Katsumata, and S. Saito, "Development Status of Terumo Implantable Left Ventricular Assist System." *Artif. Organs*, vol. 25, no.5, pp. 411–413, 2001.

[62] J. Asama, T. Shinshi, H. Hoshi, S. Takatani, and A. Shimokohbe, "A Compact Highly Efficient and Low Hemolytic Centrifugal Blood Pump with a Magnetically Levitated Impeller," *Artif. Organs*, vol. 30, no. 3, pp. 160–167, Mar. 2006.

[63] M. Morshuis, A. El-Banayosy, L. Arusoglu, R. Koerfer, R. Hetzer, G. Wieselthaler, A. Pavie, and C. Nojiri, "European Experience of DuraHeart Magnetically Levitated Centrifugal Left Ventricular Assist System," *Eur J Cardiothorac Surg*, vol. 35, no. 6, pp. 1020–1028, 2009.

[64] M. Morshuis, M. Schoenbrodt, and C. Nojiri, "DuraHeart Magnetically Levitated Centrifugal Left Ventricular Assist System for Advanced Heart Failure Patients," *Expert Rev.*, 2010.

[65] P. D. Wearden, V. O. Morell, B. B. Keller, S. a Webber, H. S. Borovetz, S. F. Badylak, J. R. Boston, R. L. Kormos, M. V Kameneva,

M. Simaan, T. a Snyder, H. Tsukui, W. R. Wagner, J. F. Antaki, C. Diao, S. Vandenberghe, J. Gardiner, C. M. Li, D. Noh, D. Paden, B. Paden, J. Wu, G. B. Bearnson, G. Jacobs, J. Kirk, P. Khanwilkar, J. W. Long, S. Miles, J. a Hawkins, P. C. Kouretas, and R. E. Shaddy, "The PediaFlow Pediatric Ventricular Assist Device," *Semin. Thorac. Cardiovasc. Surg. Pediatr. Card. Surg. Annu.*, pp. 92–98, Jan. 2006.

[66] C. Chen, B. Paden, J. Antaki, J. Ludlow, D. Paden, and R. Crowson, "A Magnetic Suspension Theory and Its Application to the HeartQuest Ventricular Assist Device," *Artif. Organs*, vol. 26, no. 11, pp. 947–951, 2002.

[67] J. M. Gardiner, J. Wu, M. D. Noh, J. F. Antaki, T. a Snyder, D. B. Paden, and B. E. Paden, "Thermal Analysis of the PediaFlow Pediatric Ventricular Assist Device," *ASAIO J.*, vol. 53, no. 1, pp. 65–73, 2007.

[68] "MiTiHeart Corporation Technical Specifications Page." [Online]. Available: http://www.mitiheart.com/#/technical-specifications/ 4556354199.

[69] Olsen, D. B., G. Bramm, and P. Novak, "Magnetically Suspended and Rotated Impellor Pump Apparatus and Method," US Patent 6015272, 1987.

[70] Antaki, J. F., B. Paden, G. Burgreen, and N. Groom, "Magnetically Suspended Miniature Fluid Pump and Method of Designing the Same," US Patent 4688998, 2000.

About the Authors

Steven Day holds a BS degree in mechanical engineering and Ph.D. in mechanical and aerospace engineering from the University of Virginia, as well as a diploma from the von Karman Institute for Fluid Dynamics. He is currently on the Mechanical Engineering faculty at the Rochester Institute of Technology. Dr. Day's research and expertise deals with the application of experimental and computational fluid mechanics to a range of applied and biological flows, including implantable blood pumps. He has worked on two magnetically levitated ventricular assist devices during the past two decades, most recently directing the engineering efforts of the LEV-VAD, an axial flow magnetically levitated implantable pump.

Shanbao Cheng holds a BS MS degree in mechanical engineering from Sichuan University, China, and Ph.D. in mechanical and aerospace engineering from Nanyang Technological University, Singapore. He did his postdoctoral research at Rochester Institute of Technology in the field of magnetically levitated blood pump and at Massachusetts Institute of Technology in the field of surgical robotics. He is currently Principle Design Engineer working at Ellipse Technologies. Dr. Cheng's research and expertise deals with the mechanical design and mechatronics application to medical devices and magnetic bearings. He has worked on two magnetically levitated ventricular assist devices during the past two decades, most recently participating the engineering efforts of the LEV-VAD, an axial flow magnetically levitated implantable pump.

Arnold David Gomez is a research associate in the Department of Electrical and Computer Engineering at the Johns Hopkins University. He earned a Ph.D. in Bioengineering from the University of Utah, and an MS in Mechanical Engineering from the Rochester institute of technology. He holds undergraduate degrees from the Rochester Institute of Technology and State University of New York. Dr. Gomez specializes on dynamic estimation using computational models and has applied his expertise in the fields of control systems including a magnetically levitated ventricular assist device, and imaging-based motion estimation of cardiovascular and brain tissue.

About the Guest Editors

Said Jahanmir is a technology leader with extensive technical and management experience in academia, US government, and industry. He is the President of Boston Tribology Associates, a unique consulting firm providing innovative friction, wear and & lubrication solutions. He has been selected as the ASME Federal Government Science and Technology Policy Fellow (2015–2016). He served as President and CEO of MiTiHeart Corporation and Vice President for biotechnology at Mohawk Innovative Technology, Inc. (2002–2015), where he lead research and development efforts on implantable blood pumps, high-temperature coatings, high-speed micro-machining and high-speed oil-free compressors. His leadership has led to the development and pre-clinical testing of a new generation of mechanical heart assist pumps with magnetic bearings for heart failure patients, and the development of a novel ultra high-speed micro-machining spindle with rotational speeds beyond 500,000 rpm. Prior to joining MiTi he was associated with the National Institute of Standards and Technology (NIST), where he served in several capacities between 1987 and 2002 including Leader of the Ceramic Manufacturing Group. He directed research activities that ranged from characterization of ceramic powders to assessment of mechanical properties of ceramics. He coordinated several international collaborations on pre-standards research that led to ASTM and ISO standards. He established and managed a joint research program between NIST, industry and academia and developed authoritative guides for machining of advanced ceramics. Among his prior experience, he was the first Director of the Tribology Program (1985–1987) at the National Science Foundation; Senior Research Engineer (1980–1985) at Exxon Research and Engineering Company; Assistant Professor of mechanical engineering (1977–1980) at Cornell University; Lecturer (1976–1977) at the University of California at Berkeley; and Instructor (1975–1976) at the Massachusetts Institute of Technology (MIT). He was an Adjunct Professor of mechanical engineering at the University Delaware (1999–2006) and served as Honorary Research Professor at Hanyang University in South Korea (1998–2002). He has been a Visiting Lecturer at MIT since 2007 teaching summer short courses in the Professional Education Program.

His pioneering research in tribology, manufacturing and medical devices is widely recognized in the scientific and engineering communities. His groundbreaking research on tribology was instrumental in establishing fundamental mechanics and materials science viewpoint for wear and provided a clear and simple understanding of the fundamentals of boundary lubrication. His research on wear and machining of advanced ceramics and dental materials resulted in a series of highly cited publications. He identified the basic mechanisms of wear and new insights into the fundamental micro-mechanisms of machining and damage formation in advanced ceramics and dental restorations. He has published more than 240 archival papers and major reports and has edited several books and conference proceedings. He has served as the founding Executive Editor of the Machining Science and Technology journal, now in its 18th year. He holds seven US and EU patents.

He received Honorary Membership in ASME in 2013, recognized for seminal contributions to the advancement of mechanical engineering, particularly the multidisciplinary technologies in tribology, manufacturing, biomedical materials and devices, and in the promotion of standards; and for significant contributions to ASME. An ASME Fellow, he has been an active volunteer in the ASME and a strong advocate for change and growth. As chair of the Tribology Division, he revised the bylaws and initiated many innovative projects. Later, as chair of the Board on Research and Technology Development and vice president for research; he streamlined the operating procedures and established fiscal management. As chair of the International Congress Committee he initiated the track-based technical program and encouraged collaboration among ASME divisions and sectors. As a governor at large (2009–2012) he served on several Board committees and Presidential task forces, and was a driving force for the ASME Global Impact Strategic Initiative and the new ASME website. He received ASME's Dedicated Service Award in 1995 and Mayo D. Hersey Award in 2001, and the Tribology Division's Donald Wilcock Distinguished Service Award in 2009.

He is a Fellow of the Society of Tribologists and Lubrication Engineers (STLE) and has served in various leadership positions. He is a former member of the American Society for Artificial Internal Organs and the International Society for Rotary Blood Pumps. Among his other honors, Jahanmir received STLE's International Award and

Honorary Membership (1997), and the Federal Laboratory Consortium's Technology Transfer Award (2000). He was elected to chair the Gordon Research Conference on Tribology (1998). He served as President of Partnership for Educational Policy (2002–2003), a new organization formed to inform the public and policy makers on educational issues that have a wide reaching impact on K-12 education and was honored as the Community Hero by the Montgomery County Civic Federation (1999) for his contribution to local educational issues. He is listed in Who's Who in America, Who's Who in Science and Engineering and American Men and Women of Science.

He received his bachelor's degree in mechanical engineering from the University of Washington and his master's degree and Ph.D. in mechanical engineering from MIT.

William Weiss is the Howard E. Morgan Professor of Surgery and Bioengineering in the College of Medicine at Pennsylvania State University in Hershey, PA. Professor Weiss's research activities are primarily related to the design, testing, and clinical application of mechanical circulatory support systems, including the Ventricular Assist Device (VAD) and Total Artificial Heart (TAH).

A major focus has been the development of completely implantable systems intended for long term support in adults. These systems present a number of engineering challenges in order to meet the requirements of long life, high reliability, small size, and energy efficiency. Dr. Weiss has pioneered the clinical use of wireless inductive power transmission as a means of eliminating infection-prone percutaneous cables. This technology was part of the first wireless VAD used in humans, as well as an implantable TAH. Other related research includes system integration, simulation, motor control, telemetry, and system testing. Recent efforts include studies to minimize device-related adverse effects, such as thrombosis, hemolysis, and acquired von Willebrand syndrome. Dr. Weiss also leads the development of a Pediatric VAD intended for infants and small children. A major challenge in developing small VADs has been minimizing thrombus formation which requires a multidisciplinary effort in fluid mechanics, hematology, and animal testing.

Conrad M. Zapanta is a Teaching Professor and the Associate Department Head in the Department of Biomedical Engineering at

Carnegie Mellon University in Pittsburgh, PA. Dr. Zapanta received his Ph.D. in Bioengineering from the Pennsylvania State University in University Park, PA, and his B.S. in Mechanical Engineering (with an option in Biomedical Engineering) from Carnegie Mellon University. Dr. Zapanta has served as a Visiting Assistant Professor of Engineering at Hope College in Holland, MI, an Adjunct Professor of Engineering at Austin Community College in Austin, TX, and as an Assistant Professor of Surgery and Bioengineering at the Pennsylvania State University in Hershey, PA. He has also worked for CarboMedics Inc. in Austin, TX, in the research and development of prosthetic heart valves.

Dr. Zapanta's primary teaching responsibilities are Biomedical Engineering Laboratory and Design. Additional teaching interests include medical device design education and professional issues in biomedical engineering. Dr. Zapanta's responsibilities as Associate Department head include overseeing the undergraduate curriculum and undergraduate student advising.

Dr. Zapanta's research interests are in developing medical devices to treat cardiovascular disease, focusing on the areas of cardiac assist devices and prosthetic heart valves.

Dr. Zapanta is an active member in the American Society for Artificial Internal Organs, American Society of Mechanical Engineers, the American Society for Engineering Education, and the Biomedical Engineering Society. He is a reviewer for several biomedical engineering journals. Dr. Zapanta also serves as a reviewer for the National Institutes of Health (NIH), Cardiovascular Sciences Small Business Special Emphasis Panel and as an ABET Program Evaluator (PEV) for Bioengineering and Biomedical Engineering programs.